Solved:
THE RIDDLE OF ILLNESS

Other Keats titles of relevant interest

Brain Allergies
by William H. Philpott, M.D. and Dwight K. Kalita, Ph.D.

How to Do Something About the Way You Feel
by David L. Messenger, M.D. with John C. Souter

Nourishing Your Child
by Ray C. Wunderlich, M.D. and Dwight K. Kalita, Ph.D.

Nutrients to Age Without Senility
by Abram Hoffer, M.D. and Morton Walker, D.P.M.

Orthomolecular Nutrition
by Abram Hoffer, M.D. and Morton Walker, D.P.M.

Physician's Handbook on Orthomolecular Medicine
by Roger J. Williams, Ph.D. and Dwight K. Kalita, Ph.D.

Trace Elements, Hair Analysis and Nutrition
by Richard A. Passwater, Ph.D. and Elmer M. Cranton, M.D.

Victory Over Diabetes
by William Philpott, M.D. and Dwight K. Kalita, Ph.D.

Solved:
THE RIDDLE OF ILLNESS

STEPHEN E. LANGER, M.D.
WITH JAMES F. SCHEER

KEATS PUBLISHING, INC.　　NEW CANAAN, CONNECTICUT

Library of Congress Cataloging in Publication Data

Langer, Stephen E.
  Solved, the riddle of illness.

  Bibliography: p.
  Includes index.
  1. Hypothyroidism—Complications and sequelae.
2. Hypothyroidism—Prevention.   3. Health.
I. Scheer, James F. II. Title.
RC657.L3 1984   616.4′44   84-12586
ISBN 0-87983-370-X
ISBN 0-87983-357-2 (pbk.)

SOLVED: THE RIDDLE OF ILLNESS

Printed in the United States of America

KEATS PUBLISHING, INC.
27 Pine Street, New Canaan, Connecticut 06840

Dedicated to my darling daughter, Caroline Viva,
my parents, Abner and Lillian,
and my brother, Stuart

CONTENTS

ACKNOWLEDGMENTS

A prime mover in clinical research on the thyroid gland for half a century, Broda O. Barnes, M.D., Ph.D. was also a prime mover behind the writing of this book, by liberally giving his time, abundant information, encouragement and inspiration to my coauthor, James F. Scheer, and me. I know of no one else in the world who has done so much as a medical doctor, writer, lecturer and talk show guest to alert millions to the often hidden causes of illness, as well as to simple ways to stay well for life.

This book is intended to carry the Barnes tradition forward—to reveal the unsuspected reasons for illness and sound ways of achieving and maintaining wellness.

Credit for encouraging the writing of *Solved: The Riddle of Illness* also goes to Mr. George Shutt, of Glendora, California, president of Shutt Medical Technologies, who for many years has served as Dr. Barnes's volunteer publicist. George has made a second career—concurrent and non-profit—of disseminating information on subnormal thyroid function. By forming a new private enterprise, he has realized funding to launch a hypothyroidism foundation to educate the public and the medical profession and to facilitate research efforts in this critically important area.

In addition, thanks go to my friend Jeffrey Bland, Ph.D., Professor of Nutritional Biochemistry at the University of Puget Sound, Director of the Bellevue Redmond Medical Laboratory and, at this writing, a visiting faculty member at the Linus Pauling Institute. I drew some of the book's material from a talk he gave when he, Dr. Barnes and I were speakers at the Webster-Barnes Foundation Conference in Dallas, Texas.

I am also grateful to William H. Philpott, M.D., from whose superb book, *Victory Over Diabetes*, I used some material with permission from Nathan Keats, president of Keats Publishing, Inc., publishers of his book and this one.

Edward R. Pinckney, M.D., and his wife Cathey, of Beverly Hills, California, prominent medical writers, generously supplied key material from several of their books and other publications for use in *Solved: The Riddle of Illness*.

Special thanks go to Carolyn Scheer for invaluable assistance in research, editing and typing of this manuscript under adverse circumstances.

All too rarely are editors given credit for contributions which are so vitally important to the quality of a book. I will not commit this sin of omission. Therefore, I salute Ellen Kapustka, associate editor at Keats Publishing, who carried out her task brilliantly.

Stephen E. Langer, M.D.

PREFACE

Solved: The Riddle of Illness is a unique book, one that has been too long in coming. It makes a landmark contribution to the recognition, prevention and management of common health disorders whose diagnoses often defy the most up-to-date medical technology and skill.

Unfortunately, doctors who have seemingly exhausted all possibilities with patients tend to put such ailments into the category of "psychosomatic" or "psychogenic," polite labels for hypochondria. Although such common symptoms as overwhelming fatigue and depression can certainly be caused by emotional problems, they are often physical in origin.

As an endocrinologist of long standing, I know from considerable experience that identification of the root cause of many physical disorders is frequently missed. Some sixty-four different symptoms are associated with one root cause—hypothyroidism—an ailment so widespread and sometimes so difficult to detect that a vast percentage of the population unknowingly suffers from it. It is a sad fact that today's medicine is less effective than it could be, because it accents the treatment of symptoms, while underlying causes go undiscovered and therefore untreated.

Dr. Langer's book probes deeply and exposes these underlying causes. In addition to his primary goal of providing information for lay people, Dr. Langer is alerting colleagues to new information and new alternatives so that they can achieve a higher percentage of cures, greater career satisfaction and—above all—greater patient satisfaction.

Today we physicians are encouraging patients to take more responsibility for their care for the very good reason that they can do a great deal more than they are doing to prevent disease and to promote robust health, the best weapon against illness.

Dr. Langer has elevated this trend to an even higher level throughout the pages of *Solved: The Riddle of Illness*. Let me cite just one of many examples. He presents a simple, do-it-yourself test that reveals the presence of a key root cause for numerous symptoms. This invaluable service is particularly welcome in this age of skyrocketing health care costs.

Among many information-packed chapters that can bring dramatic upgrading of health to readers is "Care and Feeding of the Thyroid," which contains vitally important—even critical—information that I have never before seen in a book. There might have been a time when we could take the thyroid gland for granted—not in the goiter belts, of course—but that day has passed. With the advent of processed foods and depleted soils, we cannot always be sure of being well nourished. It is important therefore to know how to keep ourselves healthy with the proper food supplements, a subject which Dr. Langer covers in depth. Particularly important is understanding how to keep the thyroid healthy so that this essential gland can help the rest of the body stay healthy.

I feel strongly that *Solved: The Riddle of Illness* deserves to be on the bookshelf of every health-conscious individual as well as on that of all medical doctors who are open to new information that can benefit their patients and themselves.

Nathan Becker, M.D.
San Francisco

Please Note!

SOLVED: THE RIDDLE OF ILLNESS suggests a way of life for reaching and maintaining peak health. It is based on the best of the latest research and the best of time-tested methods—some of the latter long forgotten.

Although the medical profession encourages us to take more responsibility for our health, seeking wellness should be done in cooperation with a doctor. More and more physicians are becoming aware of the benefits to be derived from preventive methods—among them optimum nutrition.

This book is not to be considered a prescription. You are unique. You have your own set of individual variations—physical, mental and emotional. Only the doctor who knows, examines and treats you can prescribe for you. For this reason, the authors and publishers cannot take medical or legal responsibility of having the contents of this book considered a prescription for anyone.

With regard to case studies used in this book we have made every effort to conceal the identity of all individuals in order to preserve their privacy. To this end, all names, physical descriptions and even professions have been changed.

Solved:
THE RIDDLE OF ILLNESS

1

"NOTHING ORGANICALLY WRONG"

"Dr. Langer, I hate sex!"

Tears glistened in the eyes of the attractive thirty-year-old woman seated across the desk from me.

"Maybe it's my fatigue," she continued. "Half awake, in a mental fog, I drag around the office. At home in the evening, I collapse, exhausted, when my husband wants me most. Yet how can I even think of having sex when my body cries out just for survival?"

Particularly upsetting to this patient, whom I'll call Connie, was the assessment of her condition by previous doctors: "There's nothing organically wrong."

Allison's problem was somewhat different. She enjoyed sex but usually turned off her mate with icy cold hands and feet.

Tired, drowsy, anxious, often depressed, she caught every cold that came her way, had frequent sinus and upper respiratory infections and severe headaches.

"My doctor can't find a thing wrong," she told me. "He calls me the world's foremost hypochondriac."

Eloise had no complaints about her sex life, only her sex. Difficult menstruation, which had started prematurely at age ten, caused her to miss school and, now, time from her prosperous advertising agency. To cope with exhaustion and with being cold, she drank mug after mug of hot coffee. She often experienced acute anxiety and occasional feelings of doom.

"My former doctor—and I do mean *former*—made me furious during my last office visit," she explained. "He told me, 'I advise you to take a more wholesome view of your health, because there's nothing organically wrong.'"

Like these women, Phil, a brilliant twenty-nine-year-old computer circuitry designer, had a mixed bag of problems—sudden inability to perform sexually, increasing difficulty producing innovative ideas, and minimal energy and endurance.

"My sexual failure is humiliating," he admitted, "but mental sluggishness and lack of energy are threatening my income and career. Coffee and pep pills don't do a thing for me. It's as if somebody pulled the plug on my power source."

His previous physician had tried a series of testosterone injections, which had given him only a minor charge and no improvement in his sex life or performance in business. Too young to be old, Phil was naturally dejected.

The four patients had two things in common: frustration and the same basic ailment. During their individual consultations with me, I informed them:

"Your thyroid function needs checking."

Their reactions could be summed up in the words: "Not *another* test!" All of them had gone through exhaustive tests, including one for thyroid function, at a cost of hundreds of dollars.

"This won't cost you a cent," I assured them. "You can do the Barnes Basal Temperature Test yourself at home."

They were puzzled. Who had ever heard of a no-cost test? Then I explained how to do it.

"Before going to bed tonight, shake down a thermometer.

Leave it on the bedside table. As soon as you wake up in the morning after a good night's sleep—no later—tuck the thermometer snugly in your armpit for ten minutes as you lie there.

"If your thyroid function is normal, your temperature should be in the range from 97.8 to 98.2 degrees Fahrenheit. If it's lower, you are probably hypothyroid—your thyroid gland is under-functioning—and your physical problems and related ones have probably been caused or at least influenced by that. The test should be done on two consecutive days."

To the women, I said, "You get the most accurate readings if you're not menstruating (temperature fluctuates at this time) or on the second or third days of menstruation."

Reported results confirmed my suspicions: all were indeed hypothyroid. The treatment—natural desiccated thyroid supplement—brought gratifying results: freedom from their ailments in less than two months. Eloise was ecstatic about painless menstruation and normal body temperature. Appreciative husbands of Connie and Allison told me that thyroid had saved their sex life and marriage. Phil went even further. He said, "It saved my whole life."

Over sixteen years as a medical doctor, I have been privileged to help many Connies, Allisons, Eloises and Phils. In fact, I seem to specialize in patients whose symptoms are not readily diagnosed—persons who have been through the traditional system and possibly have been rejected as psychosomatic cases or as hypochondriacs.

A graduate of the New York College of Medicine at Buffalo, I spent some time studying medical psychology before realizing that I couldn't accept one of the basic assumptions of traditional Western allopathic medicine—the sharp cleavage between mind and body. I was troubled that patients should be branded as "psychological problems" or as having "psychogenic problems," as opposed to having "ailments of the body." It seemed that the twain would never meet.

In my frame of reference, mind and body are two expressions of the same thing. As I moved out of medical psychology, I realized another key fact about my professional stance. I couldn't build a shrine before the double-blind approach so highly revered in medical schools. It is certainly valid, but it is just one belief system among many. Belief systems should be used pragmatically, not be regarded as sacred. They should be continually transcended if something better comes along—even if that something doesn't fit into the tidy training mold of medical doctors.

Because of this position, I can draw upon the best of today's medicine and still think and act independently. Therefore, if patients have no clinical findings to back up a laundry list of complaints, I don't automatically conclude that they are hypochondriacs, neurotics or psychotics. After an examination and the taking of a thorough history (which may not reveal reasons for their problems), I still do not paste a negative label on them. After all, no medical system or doctor is infallible. Often there is a physical basis for many symptoms, a cause not always apparent within the framework of traditional clinical medicine.

One major basis frequently overlooked is hypothyroidism—under-functioning of the thyroid gland. Even a seemingly slight deficiency in thyroid hormone can cause an incredible number and variety of sabotaging physical, emotional and mental ailments.

For the benefit of my patients and the expansion of my professional horizons, I am thankful that I stumbled across the monumental research in this area of Broda O. Barnes, M.D., Ph.D., one of the world's foremost authorities on the thyroid gland. This wealth of information revolutionized my practice of preventive health maintenance more than any other single factor.

Speaking from almost fifty years of clinical experimentation, Dr. Barnes stated that no less than 40 percent of the adult population of the United States suffers from an often hidden condition known as hypothyroidism. In medical school we saw a few cases, but no one paid much attention to them. The 40 percent figure struck me as a gross exaggeration until I followed the Barnes method in my practice and found the percentage running slightly higher.

Lecturing to physicians and lay people worldwide, Dr. Barnes warned that serious hypothyroidism was going virtually undetected, because of doctors' almost total reliance upon laboratory blood tests. Why should millions suffer needlessly from the insidious effects of hypothyroidism when a simple, accurate thyroid function test was available to everyone? After all, his underarm test had been painstakingly checked for accuracy against basal metabolism results in thousands of persons in the late 1930s and early 1940s and a paper on the subject had been published in one of the most prestigious medical journals.

Initially, I couldn't buy the idea of downgrading the value of blood tests. The scientist in me said that Dr. Barnes, for some unknown reason, was trying to break the back of traditional clinical medicine. Yet at the same time his hypothesis attracted me. Why not give it a fair trial?

Obviously, Dr. Barnes was not out to sell something, because thyroid hormone is one of the cheapest substances on the market. He did not claim that an underactive thyroid was the sole cause of a host of ailments, only that it played a role in them, and that many traditional treatments for chronic degenerative diseases would not work smoothly—or at all—until the thyroid gland was properly tested, and, if necessary, supplemented. Certainly he never claimed that thyroid hormone was a panacea.

About this time, I began appearing as a guest on television and radio talk shows, as well as conducting my own question and answer radio show in the San Francisco area, and I set up a phone interview with Dr. Barnes, then practicing medicine in Fort Collins, Colorado. For two hours, Dr. Barnes answered my questions and those from the audience so directly, factually and convincingly, that I was prompted to take my own basal temperature; I found it somewhat low. Shortly after I started using a small daily dosage of natural desiccated thyroid supplement, remarkable changes occurred: my energy shot up, my ability to concentrate improved dramatically and many minor nagging symptoms disappeared.

Then I judiciously began using the Barnes Basal Temperature Test on a number of problem patients and, when it was indicated, prescribed the thyroid supplement. Their quick, positive response made me a believer. Soon I found that this test is the key to treating a number of chronic degenerative illnesses that I couldn't touch by conventional methods. I learned what most doctors know: that there is always a population of people who defy many of our best clinical approaches. My surprise was in seeing how large that population is.

Unusual success and satisfaction with Dr. Barnes's methods

stirred up questions in my mind. How did he discover that temperature is a more reliable indicator of thyroid function than the pride of modern medical technology, lab tests? How did he learn that even slight hypothyroidism—often not detectable by conventional measuring devices or systems—can cause or contribute to serious ailments in women, men and children?

Once I became well acquainted with Dr. Barnes, I learned firsthand the fascinating facts which have helped me treat the neglected gland of hundreds of patients in a proper manner so that they could become revitalized. Here is how he tells it:

In the early 1930s, even before planning to become a physician, I was assigned to study the thyroid gland for my doctorate in physiology at the University of Chicago, under Dr. Anton J. Carlson, a giant in the field.

Soon I had a Ph.D. after my name, and Dr. Carlson assigned me to teach endocrinology to future physicians. One of my duties was to show a motion picture to demonstrate the powerful influence of the thyroid gland on every living cell of every body system.

Students were shocked at the rapid deterioration of a small rabbit after removal of its thyroid. Previously warm at room temperature, active and alert, the animal now shivered with cold, moved in slow motion, drugged with fatigue—as if old and feeble. Its fur was dry, its skin was scaly, its mucous membranes were infected—particularly in the respiratory system—and its heartbeat and muscles were weak. My respect for the tiny thyroid gland increased with every class.

Striving to increase my effectiveness as an instructor, I completed the medical curriculum, not realizing that I would soon do more doctoring than teaching. Upon completion of my internship in 1937, I took the Hippocratic oath, and the philosophy of Hippocrates, the Father of Greek medicine, is still branded on my brain, particularly the following statement:

"It is not to be expected that he should know the remedies of illnesses who knows not their origin."

Treating the symptoms, the usual approach in modern medicine, was not enough. I wanted to probe to the roots of illnesses, to causes. Now, licensed to practice, I had an immediate opportunity.

Charlotte, my wife, who developed tuberculosis, became my first patient. Galen, the celebrated physician of the second century, had said, "If you develop tuberculosis, go to the mountains and buy a cow."

We did both, settling in the then clean-air countryside near Denver, where we not only drank fresh milk but picked and ate ripe vegetables and fruit from our garden and trees. Charlotte and I took a small amount of thyroid daily to compensate for hypothyroidism. Her rapid recovery and my boundless energy and endurance demonstrated the value of natural, nutrient-packed food—a major part of the foundation for good health—and thyroid supplementation.

Lessons learned from the rabbit helped with my first paying patient, a clubwoman who had complained of female problems, coldness, lack of energy, anxiety, low blood pressure and one infection after another. She had been thoroughly examined and treated in a world-renowned midwestern clinic, where no physical reason for her symptoms could be found.

"Doctor, I spent a small fortune there and came away with no satisfaction. What makes me indignant is that they think I'm a hypochondriac."

I put her on a daily grain of natural thyroid extract and she soon improved, recovering completely in seven weeks.

That rabbit continued to make me look good. This grateful woman sent me friends who had one or more similar complaints with no apparent measurable causes: sexual dysfunction, little or no sensation in the vagina, feeling cold, excruciating menstrual pain (then commonly treated with aspirin and bedrest), too frequent periods, too copious blood flow, acute headaches, fatigue, irritability, hair-trigger temper and infections (mainly in the vaginal and urinary channels).

Small doses of natural desiccated thyroid improved or eliminated these conditions. Husbands began coming to me. Spectacular recoveries of women and men enlightened and puzzled me. Surely so many of my patients would not have been helped by thyroid if it had not been necessary. Yet other doctors had given them comprehensive physical exams, including a basal metabolism test (the then accepted measurement of thyroid function), without detecting hypothyroidism. Could it be that thyroid deficiency too slight to be recorded contributed to or caused many illnesses? Could the basal metabolism test be so far wrong that it actually concealed hypothyroidism? Could known symptoms of low thyroid function be a more reliable indicator than the basal metabolism test?

Searching for answers—even clues—I paged through countless

journals in the Denver Medical Library and found a revealing, detailed description of the first acute hypothyroid patient who had symptoms similar to those of my patients, though far more exaggerated.

In 1877 Dr. William N. Ord, a brilliant London clinician, had made a milestone discovery while performing an autopsy on a mature woman. Medical records disclosed that she had been constantly cold and exhausted, prone to fall asleep if not moving around, incapable of thinking or speaking without extreme effort, unable to sew because of numb and clumsy hands, inclined to suffer frequent headaches and menopausal problems, as well as infections and a kidney ailment causing bloody urine.

He was fascinated by her unsightly physical degeneration—a moon face too swollen to change expression (a feature of cretinism) and body skin and connective tissue bloated with fluid. When Dr. Ord cut into her skin, expecting water to run off (as in kidney failure), a thick, glue-like substance called mucin remained fixed there. To give a name to this condition, he took the Greek word for mucin, "myx," and wedded it to "edema," the description for water-logged tissue, calling it "myxedema."

The woman's arteries showed advanced atherosclerosis. Coronary, kidney and brain arteries were almost clogged. He was amazed at the sight of the woman's thyroid gland, so overgrown and choked with fibrous tissue that it had stopped functioning. He concluded that this was what had caused myxedema and atherosclerosis.

Mulling over the woman's list of symptoms, I found six common denominators in my far milder cases of hypothyroidism: subnormal temperature, fatigue, drowsiness, depression, female problems and infections.

Despite exhaustive study of the thyroid gland, I still thought it incredible that this tiny, lightweight (less than an ounce), coral-colored bow-tie semi-circling the windpipe under the Adam's apple could be so critical to living and to the quality of life. Yet numerous well-designed experiments had already shown that production of thyroid hormone can make or break a person's health.

All of your blood—approximately five quarts—circulates through the thyroid gland once every hour, bringing iodide, the material your thyroid needs to make hormones, as well as a hormone from the anterior pituitary gland to stimulate production from the thyroid. Your thyroid also stores and discharges thyroid hormone into the bloodstream for delivery to your cells where and when needed.

Too little thyroid hormone (in hypothyroidism) causes your motor to run sluggishly. Heartbeat slows, blood pressure drops, circulation becomes lazy (contributing to discomfort from cold, particularly in the hands and feet), energy and endurance are low, digestion slows down, constipation is common, headaches occur frequently, hair becomes lifeless and falls out more readily, nails are brittle, wounds heal slowly, thinking is slow, memory undependable and sex urge weak or dormant. The effects of hypothyroidism are felt in each of your trillions of cells in every organ and tissue of your body.

Too much thyroid hormone, in hyperthyroidism, makes your motor race; heartbeat increases, blood pressure rises, blood volume swells; you flush from overheating, often to the level of a mild fever; you perspire profusely, are nervous and sleepless, and you may have diarrhea. (Similar symptoms may occur if a hypothyroid is given too much thyroid supplement.)

Teamwork of the thyroid and pituitary glands in infants, children and youths encourages growth of the skeleton and sexual organs, contributes to eruption of teeth and development of the brain.

One of the most succinct and colorful summations of the dramatic function of the thyroid (which I happened upon considerably later) is in the writings of endocrinologist Herman H. Rubin, M.D.: "... a few grains of thyroid may be the main difference between a captain of industry and the office boy who is always dragging his feet."[1] Then he added that a close and sympathetic relationship exists between the thyroid and sex glands of men and women, that sexual function really is an expression of energy. Due to the fact the thyroid is the governor of our uses of energy, we shouldn't be too surprised by the association. Alertness, animation, fire and sparkle result from a properly functioning thyroid. These qualities show themselves particularly in glamor and sexual attractiveness.

In my reading, I came across another succinct summary on the critical importance of the thyroid gland by the late Louis Berman, M.D., world-renowned endocrinologist:

"Without thyroid, there can be no complexity of thought, no learning, no education, no habit formation, no responsive energy for situations as well as no physical unfolding of faculty and function. No reproduction of kind with no sign of adolescence at expected age and no exhibition of sex tendencies thereafter."[2]

With no thyroid gland, you and I would not be human at all—we'd be vegetables!

In a continuing search of the literature, I noticed that subnormal temperature appeared to be a common denominator in hypothyroidism. Many decades of pioneering research in England had demonstrated that if metabolism is low, temperature is also low. Each hypothyroid patient who came to my office was a verification of this fact.

Could temperature give a more accurate indication of hypothyroidism than the basal metabolism test? I decided to find out. In my private practice and, later, as professor of Health Education at the University of Denver, I took the oral temperature of hundreds of male and female patients and students and also gave them the basal metabolism test, making sure that no subjects had an infection, which would have caused a false reading.

I then compared results of both measurements with known symptoms of hypothyroidism and learned that temperature was the more accurate indicator by far.

In a subsequent study of 1,000 college students, reported in the August, 1942, issue of *Journal of the American Medical Association*, I again found that the relationship of subnormal temperature to accepted major symptoms of hypothyroidism was significantly greater than to basal metabolism readings.

Dr. Joseph Ehrlich and I, while U.S. Army medical officers in Kingman, Arizona, during World War II, refined the test, taking oral, rectal and armpit temperatures of 1,000 soldiers. We found that, barring sore throats, sinusitis or colds, which raise oral temperature, mouth and armpit temperatures are nearly identical.

Out of these experiments came the Barnes Basal Temperature Test, which, for many years, has been listed in the Physicians Desk Reference (the PDR). Many physicians now rely on this test because by using it they have discovered tens of thousands of hypothyroid individuals who were rated normal by conventional tests. But even though the temperature test's accuracy has been abundantly demonstrated, we do not lean exclusively on its results. We verify them with classical symptoms of hypothyroidism and the patient's thorough medical history, carefully correlating and interpreting data.

Any less painstaking procedure can lead to possible error. A Mayo Clinic study by Drs. Joseph C. Scott, Jr. and Elizabeth Mussey made this point clearly when they found that a patient · can be regarded as mildly hypothyroid by one physician and normal by another, based on results of just one office interview or test. "No single test or procedure will define the status of the thyroid gland," they write. "Further, any combination of methods may lead to erroneous interpretation or to inconsistent results. The clinician must have the faculty of correlating the clinical appearance of the patient with laboratory findings."[3]

Despite the validity of this position, present-day doctors, enchanted by the laboratory test, often make it the sole and final authority. Is this wise or otherwise?

You be the judge.

The Center for Disease Control routinely sends out specimens to 980 licensed laboratories—some 7 percent of all laboratories in the United States. Between 8 and 25 percent of the tests yield erroneous results, according to an article in *American Medical News*.[4] These labs process all kinds of tests, including critical ones for thyroid function.

Edward R. Pinckney, M.D., former associate editor of the *Journal of the American Medical Association*, wrote an earth-shaking article for the *Archives of Internal Medicine* on the accuracy of medical testing. It says, in part: "... Hardly a week goes by when the FDA [Food and Drug Administration] does not recall several in-use laboratory reagents that are contaminated, defective, or inaccurately labeled. Other surveys have reported that one out of every two sphgymomanometers [the common blood-pressure checking device] gave erroneous readings, that thousands of ECG [electrocardiogram] machines were found to be improperly calibrated, and that hundreds of X-ray machines, often operated by inadequately trained technicians, were producing thousands of useless roentgenograms [X rays]."[5]

Dr. Pinckney reveals that in an American Medical Association survey, three out of four doctors admitted ordering X rays, ECGs and a multitude of laboratory and other procedures for the sole purpose of having a better defense in the event of a malpractice suit.

"The American College of Physicians is in the throes of evaluating the usefulness of medical tests," writes Dr. Pinckney. "To date, it has declared some fifty tests to be of no proven value, unreliable or obsolete."

Admitting that medical journals are constantly reporting controversy, confusion and contradictions about the significance of tests, Dr. Pinckney advocates the old-fashioned approach to doctoring: comparing results of medical tests against the physician's clinical judgment. If the doctor doesn't do this, what good are his or her training and experience?

"In three separate but similar studies, one conducted at the Mayo Clinic, the physician's history and physical examination detected twice as many alcoholics as did detailed laboratory data," writes Dr. Pinckney.

As early as 1959, a nationally recognized authority on the thyroid gland, Dr. A. S. Jackson, had published a paper in the *Journal of the American Medical Association*, declaring that low thyroid function is the most common disease entering the doctor's office and the diagnosis most missed.[6] The situation is much the same today, except that there are more tests, more misdiagnoses and more people.

Like Drs. Jackson and Barnes, I continue to see numerous previously undetected cases of hypothyroidism. For this reason, it was no surprise to learn that biochemist Roger J. Williams, discoverer of pantothenic acid (one of the B vitamins), says: "There are doubtless a great many people who are mildly deficient in thyroid hormone and would be benefited by taking it orally but are not ill enough to see a physician."[7]

The findings of Dr. James C. Wren, reported in the *Journal of the American Geriatric Society*, bear out those of Dr. Williams, as well as those of Drs. Barnes and Jackson.[8] In a five-year research project with 347 atherosclerotic patients—174 women and 173 men—only thirty-one were shown by laboratory tests to be hypothyroid. Yet when thyroid supplements were given to all subjects, measurable improvement was shown in a significant number of patients. Further, their mortality rate was less than half that of the run of this category of untreated patients. Why were results of thyroid treatment apparent across the board if only thirty-one subjects—9 percent—were hypothyroid according to conventional laboratory tests? (Later chapters will offer additional revealing data on how hypothyroidism relates to heart and artery diseases.)

A nationally known physician and author, New York City-based H. L. Newbold, M.D., who has successfully used the Barnes Basal Temperature Test for years, agrees with Dr. Barnes in his book, *Dr. Newbold's Revolutionary New Discoveries about Weight Loss*, that many people have borderline or subnormal thyroid output and can enhance their health with modest amounts of thyroid supplement.[9]

In an article, "Hypothyroidism: A Treacherous Masquerader" (*Acute Care Medicine*, May, 1984, pages 34–36), Dr. Gerald S.

Levey, an endocrinologist and chief of medicine at the University of Pittsburgh School of Medicine, warns that hypothyroidism is often such an extremely subtle disease that physicians can misinterpret its symptoms.

The correct diagnosis is often missed, because a broad range of symptoms is not generally associated with hypothyroidism, he says: severe muscle cramps, particularly at night; persistent low back pain; blood abnormalities (easy bruising, minor bleeding, heavy blood loss in menstruation, and anemia); excessive blood uric acid; stiffness of joints (mild arthritis) and a decrease in heart contractility.

These conditions can be improved or relieved by thyroid hormone therapy, he says. Dr. Levey feels that the traditional routine screening for thyroid function may not be worth the money, inasmuch as many factors—among them drugs and certain systemic states—can distort results of such tests.

Various researchers have estimated that one-fourth of the United States population is hypothyroid—considerably under the 40-plus percentage of my new patients.

You may be among them.

Now, however, you don't have to wonder whether you are or aren't. You can gather the evidence through the Barnes Basal Temperature Test, a careful review of your medical history and a check of your symptoms against the following telltale physical and emotional signs: (1) weakness; (2) dry, coarse skin; (3) lethargy; (4) slow speech; (5) swelling of face and eyelids; (6) coldness and cold skin; (7) diminished sweating; (8) thick tongue; (9) coarse hair; (10) pale skin; (11) constipation; (12) gain in weight; (13) loss of hair; (14) labored, difficult breathing; (15) swollen feet; (16) hoarseness; (17) loss of appetite; (18) excessive and/or painful menstruation; (19) nervousness; (20) heart palpitation; (21) brittle nails; (22) slow movement; (23) poor memory; (24) emotional instability; (25) depression; and (26) headaches.

If your temperature, medical history and symptoms indicate that you are hypothyroid, report to your doctor with the facts and request treatment. Most physicians are now familiar with Dr. Barnes's method of treatment and his extensive list of publications in medical journals.

It is not my intention to indicate that additional thyroid hormone is a cure-all for anything or everything that might ail you. This would be simplistic, narrow and possibly inaccurate, ignoring many other considerations, including biological and biochemical differences which make you and me individuals with varying needs.

What I am saying is that a broad and serious blind spot exists today in physical diagnosis, one that needs immediate recognition. The purpose of this book is to serve as a newly ground, polished set of lenses to bring all parts of this area sharply into our visual field.

Awareness of widespread hypothyroidism and the three-way approach to its accurate diagnosis will enable you to do one of two things: rule it out entirely or get proper treatment for it. This condition is too important to go ignored and untreated. It only worsens. Remember that the thyroid—the neglected gland—can have a mild to profound effect on every aspect of living: energy, endurance, body heat, sexuality, mind and emotions, resistance to colds and other respiratory ailments, condition of hair, skin and nails, as well as protection against diabetes and diabetic complications, heart and artery diseases and cancer. It affects how long and how well you live!

2

WHY SO MUCH HIDDEN
HYPOTHYROIDISM?

*O*ften patients, viewers of my *Medicine Man* TV program or readers of my newspaper column, ask, "How can hypothyroidism possibly be so widespread with iodized salt available to everyone?"

An important question deserves a good answer.

Iodized salt was never intended to prevent hypothyroidism, just one manifestation of it: goiter, enlargement of the thyroid gland on the front and sides of the neck. It would not be practical or healthful for us to increase salt use in an effort to get all the iodine necessary to assure normal thyroid function. Overuse of salt is implicated in a host of ailments—insomnia, obesity, stomach ulcers, edema, high blood pressure and heart disease, among others.

The daily Recommended Dietary Allowance (RDA) of iodine is 100 micrograms (mcg) for women and 120 mcg for men, although up to ten times that amount has not produced toxic effects in persons with a normal thyroid. Residents of Japan thrive on nearly 4,000 times as much iodine as Americans, all from large amounts of seafood, kelp, dulse and sea lettuce. (Warning: it could be hazardous to health, if not fatal, to ingest so much iodine in organic form.)

Goiter, premature grey hair and symptoms of hypothyroidism are rare in Japan. Is it any wonder? Much of the nation's population lives near the coast, and both soil and water are iodine-rich at or near seashores. So are vegetables, fruit and grains grown there, as well as readily accessible seafood and ocean plants.

Although we require only a minute quantity of iodine for our thyroid gland, the world's goiter belts supply just one-seventh of that amount. Goiter belts are found in mountainous or inland regions, such as the Alps, Carpathian and Pyrenees mountains of Europe, the Himalayas of Asia, the Andes mountains of South America and various parts of North America, including the valley of the St. Lawrence River, the Appalachian mountains, the Great Lakes basin and westward through Minnesota, South and North Dakota, Montana, Wyoming (and adjoining areas of Canada), the Rocky Mountains and into the northwest (parts of Oregon, Washington and British Columbia).

Over the course of many centuries, soils of mountain and inland areas become iodine-bankrupt because rain washes this trace mineral away into streams and, eventually, into the oceans. Low iodine content in the soil, however, is not the sole reason for subnormal thyroid function. Another weighty factor is inheritance. Several studies show that goiters and hypothyroidism without goiters run in families, many of whose members are hypersensitive even to minute iodine lack. Individuals prone to hypothyroidism are often revealed to have subnormal thyroid function, despite what appears to be an adequate intake of iodine.

Why did 7 percent of 8,000 school children with adequate iodine intake, surveyed in the early 1970s in Georgia, Kentucky, Michigan and Texas, have goiters? Why did the 1968 to 1970 study of individuals in ten states—from California to Massachusetts—by the Center for Disease Control end up with almost the same results? Again, more than 99 percent of those surveyed reported an acceptable intake of iodine.

A research project by Eduardo Gaitan of the Veterans Administration Medical Center and University of Mississippi Medical School, Jackson, leads him to believe region-specific environmental factors are often to blame. Returning to his native Colombia, South America, he studied this problem in the Cauca-Patia Valley area of the Andes Mountains.[1] In 1948, more than half of all school children there had goiters. The correct amount of iodine was added to the daily diet, but a 1978 survey revealed that 15 percent of the population still had goiters. Gaitan wanted to know why within this 800-kilometer-long valley the goiter incidence ranged from 1 percent to 42 percent.

His investigation permitted him to rule out insufficient iodine intake, other dietary shortcomings and socio-economic factors. "It is certain chemicals in the water supply," he told an American Chemical Society meeting in Seattle, and elaborated his reasons for this belief. He had found a high goiter area and a low goiter area in Candelaria, a non-industrial city in the Andes with a population of 8,000. This confused him until he learned that two different wells supplied the sections. Gaitan had water samples analyzed by an impartial testing laboratory, and the chemical culprits emerged in water from the high goiter district—10 to 100 parts per million of resorcinol and phthalate esters. Resorcinol has a documented reputation as a goiter-causative. The phthalate esters (normally added to various plastics to give them flexibility) also contain substances which encourage goiters. No resorcinol and negligible amounts of phthalates could be found in the water samples from the low goiter area.

What puzzled Gaitan is how resorcinol and phthalates could enter the water supply, inasmuch as they are common products of the industrial world, and Candelaria has no industry. Pipes from the well with the high level of contaminants were not made of plastics and plastic containers were not used in gathering or storing water samples. Gaitan finally concluded that these chemicals came from organic soil constituents 200 feet down.

For self-protection, it would be well for us to avoid or minimize our consumption of beverages stored in plastic containers and to check with officials of our municipal water supply to make sure it does not have a harmful content of resorcinol or phthalate esters from industrial wastes.

While Gaitan's findings may well apply to previously unexplained goiter prevalence in areas amply supplied with iodine, individual variation in size and capability of thyroid glands may also play a big part.

Dr. Roger J. Williams, whose studies on the size and functional variation of human organs have revolutionized physiology and biochemistry, writes in his book *Free and Unequal* that, among what are called normal individuals, thyroid glands vary in weight from 8 grams to 50 grams. Undoubtedly size and activity of one's thyroid gland make a difference.[2] Heredity is also an important factor.

One would have thought it possible that, in the course of several generations, marriages between hypothyroids and persons with normal thyroids would decrease hypothyroids in the population. Actually, there appear to be few such intermarriages, as many physicians conversant with problems of the thyroid have observed. Hypothyroids usually attract other hypothyroids for a basic reason: they have low energy and high sleep requirements in common. Even when short, impulsive courtships bring hypothyroids and those with normal thyroids to the altar, these couples soon realize their glaring energy mismatch and, in time, may end up in the divorce court.

In my early days of prescribing thyroid, I discovered it was a serious mistake to treat just one person of a hypothyroid couple. One of my patients was a pudgy, sluggish, no-energy man who hardly made it through a work day, mechanically munched a TV dinner with an equally dragged-out wife, then collapsed heavily into a sexless bed. A daily grain of thyroid and a diet without junk foods brought about a remarkable change in him in less than three months. He lost weight, gained energy, slept less and began going out at night, insisting that his weary wife join him in going to parties and attending concerts and the theater. Their contrasting energy levels triggered repeated quarrels. Rather than let them live unhappily ever after, I insisted that the wife take her basal temperature. Learning that it was way below par, I prescribed natural desiccated thyroid. Now this couple has made new breakthroughs in marital harmony.

The growing population of persons with subnormal thyroid

glands is not entirely due, however, to the procreation of hypothyroid couples. Medical ingenuity has something to do with it. Antibiotics have made hypothyroids less susceptible to infectious diseases which in years past would have annihilated them. Less than a century ago, almost 50 percent of all children died before becoming adults. Only those who could resist infectious diseases survived. At that time, medical science contributed little to the ability to survive. Today, over and above those who are normally infection-resistant, there is a new population segment— hypothyroids with low resistance to infectious diseases, who are kept alive by the physician's arsenal of antibiotics.

Dr. Barnes draws a sharp focus on the historic battle to survive in pointing out that humanity is constantly threatened by a grim competition of diseases: "Smallpox led the pack for many years, wiping out babies and children. Then an obscure physician, Edward Jenner, discovered that smallpox could be prevented by vaccination. Soon the champion killer was dethroned, and a larger segment of the population could live longer. Then a new menace moved in, tuberculosis, which, for more than two generations, decimated young adults, until bedrest, improved diet and, particularly, antibiotics knocked it out. Again, life expectancy rose, making the biggest advance in medical history. One disease or another keeps proving our mortality. Due to our longer life through the conquest of many infectious diseases, another killer has now claimed the championship—heart and circulatory ailments," he says.

Like Dr. Barnes, other medical doctors, clinical researchers and scientists over more than eight decades have found that thyroid supplements have won skirmishes, battles, even wars, against myriad ailments in addition to the so-called hypochondriacal conditions: fatigue, physical and sexual coldness, infectious diseases, every kind of female problem, emotional illnesses, migraine headaches, skin abnormalities, heart disease, arthritis, diabetic complications and cancer.

It is time for medical researchers and doctors to take a fresh look at the thyroid—the neglected gland—at present laboratory tests for thyroid function and at treatment of its subnormal function.

Often I am asked by patients or audiences why, if they are revealed to be hypothyroid, they cannot correct their condition simply by supplying more iodine to their thyroid gland through seafood or kelp. Sometimes they can. In first generation hypothyroidism, such compensation often proves helpful. However, in most cases, hypothyroidism has persisted for generations, so iodine supplementation may be too little, too late. This is not my finding alone. Dr. Barnes and more than one hundred of his physician followers have discovered the same phenomenon. Through experience, we have discovered that natural desiccated thyroid supplement helps make sure that enough thyroid hormone is available. It takes less than 1/100,000 ounce of this substance to keep us healthy.

A common-sense approach now assists doctors in administering thyroid supplement safely and effectively. The fear of prescribing it, so prevalent from the start of this century to the 1940s, is slowly disappearing. The secret is to balance the amount of the supplement with the amount of hormone secreted by the thyroid gland, so that an oversupply does not lull the gland into complacency and stop it from working. When the blood level of thyroid hormone drops below normal, the hypothalamus gland in the brain senses this and discharges thyroid releasing hormone (TRH). TRH influences the pituitary, the boss of the glandular company, to release thyroid stimulating hormone (TSH), which tells the thyroid to get to work. Once sufficient thyroid hormone has been produced, the pituitary puts the thyroid gland on hold.

A thyroid whose function is limited by lack of iodine, by a hereditary flaw, a tumor or some other defect can't carry out the orders of the pituitary gland. Then it needs help from the outside.

When the subnormal working of the thyroid results from the gland itself, this is called primary hypothyroidism. When underproduction is caused by imperfect function of the hypothalamus or the pituitary gland, this is called secondary hypothyroidism. Both kinds usually respond to thyroid hormone supplementation.

I start hypothyroid patients with a moderate daily dose of natural thyroid—¼ to ½ grain of Armour desiccated thyroid preparation—and increase their dosage in ¼ to ½ grain increments every seven to ten days until I obtain a dosage that achieves desired clinical results.

Usually, a child under three requires no more than ¼ grain

until he or she reaches age six, at which time ½ grain is most frequently the optimal amount needed. Teenagers generally work up to a full grain, and adults can go as high as several grains. I monitor patients carefully. If their temperature moves to normal and other symptoms begin to disappear, I keep them at this level. If not, I move them up in ¼ to ½ grain increments. In rare instances, temperature does not rise as high as normal, and additional thyroid may bring on symptoms of hyperthyroidism.

I also advise that patients take vitamin B-rich brewer's yeast along with thyroid supplement—five tablets for children and ten for teenagers and adults—since according to the theory of Murray Israel, M.D., a pioneer in thyroidology, B vitamins better equip the body to deal with outside hormones. Oxidation is speeded up by the thyroid hormones, and the B vitamins are essential to efficient transport of oxygen inside the cells. Originally, Dr. Barnes used thyroid hormones alone—with success—but, impressed by Dr. Israel's results, he added brewer's yeast to his treatment.

Dr. Israel's career in recognizing and managing widespread, unsuspected hypothyroidism also helped focus my attention on this much-neglected area of medicine. Startling results with his first case in 1934, as described at the 1966 annual meeting of the American College of Endocrinology and Nutrition, left an indelible impression on me.[3]

Called in to treat an elderly woman so far gone that her family had brought in a priest to administer the last rites, Dr. Israel found her breathing shallow, heart sounds faint, blood pressure high, coronary artery severely atherosclerotic and hypothyroidism pronounced. She had stark white hair and her pale face was flecked with dead skin. Fresh out of internship, Dr. Israel had a critical decision to make. From the standpoint of conventional medicine, the woman had two incompatible conditions, atherosclerosis and hypothyroidism. The usual treatment was to remove the thyroid gland surgically. The easy way out would have been to do nothing, but Dr. Israel decided to do something. Surgery would only make her hypothyroidism worse, so he administered 10 milligrams of thyroid along with brewer's yeast three times daily. (Brewer's yeast was then the best available vitamin B-complex source.)

He continued this regime, and in a few days, the patient turned the corner. Within two weeks, she was mentally alert and perky and walked to church. Soon her dead, pale skin peeled off, leaving her complexion pink and smooth. Black strands of hair eventually began to replace some of the white. She lived actively and enthusiastically for another twenty years.

This milestone case set a pattern of treatment for Dr. Israel, which, over the course of many years, he used successfully in over a thousand similar cases. In addition to alerting modern medicine to a more effective approach for managing coronary atherosclerosis and hypothyroidism, his triumphs spared patients with these ailments the harmful, unnecessary and costly removal of the thyroid gland and showed doctors that judicious supplementation with natural desiccated thyroid can be helpful *and* safe.

What excited Dr. Israel particularly was that the thyroid treatment had an apparent rejuvenative effect on patients. These results also intrigued a young medical doctor, Nathan Masor, who later joined Dr. Israel's research staff. After injecting Dr. Israel's formula into elderly atherosclerotic patients each week for a month, along with supplements of vitamins C and B-complex, he noticed marked physical and emotional improvement: more energy, faster movements, more endurance, better sleep and less irritability, anxiety and depression.

Encouraged, Dr. Masor did additional research, eventually concluding that organic and functional diseases are intertwined, showing two basic manifestations—fatigue and anxiety—which, in turn, cause myriad satellite symptoms, among them headache, hot flashes, depression, drowsiness, insomnia, irritability, loss of memory, inability to concentrate, impotence, guilt and inferiority feelings.

In his book *The New Psychiatry*, Dr. Masor states that symptoms of hypochondria can mimic those of any organic disease, that when fatigue and anxiety begin to disappear, so do satellite symptoms in varying degrees.[4] He explained his thyroid-vitamin therapy to the Second International Congress for Psychiatry in Zurich, Switzerland.

Dr. Masor is skeptical about the accuracy and helpfulness of the usual laboratory tests for thyroid function and asks if it isn't possible that such modern tests are incapable of detecting every case of malfunctioning thyroid gland. "This is strongly suspected in the condition of metabolic insufficiency (hypothyroidism)," he says, "wherein all tests prove normal, but the individual may suffer from a fully developed fatigue and anxiety state."[5]

On the same subject, Dr. Israel's findings are even more decisive than those of his protege. In almost forty years of practice, studies and experimentation at the Vascular Research Foundation in New York, which he founded, he observed that laboratory tests failed to uncover even a minute fraction of hypothyroids.[6] Standard tests indicated that 85 percent of his patients had normal thyroid function. Yet all of them showed marked and consistent benefits from thyroid supplementation, including comfortable body temperature and increased energy and vitality.

With so much undiagnosed hypothyroidism, it is no wonder that patients with legitimate emotional, mental and physical symptoms are sometimes written off as hypochondriacs and, even worse, left untreated, living fractional lives.

3

CARE AND FEEDING OF
THE THYROID

*D*on't take your thyroid gland for granted! Even if it is now normal, it may not stay that way unless properly fed, as one of my patients learned.

Mark's subnormal temperature, symptoms and medical history indicated hypothyroidism.

"How can that be?" He was genuinely surprised. "I take kelp tablets for iodine."

Mark had been a vegetarian for a few years, eating raw and lightly cooked vegetables, with an emphasis on carrots, sweet potatoes, spinach, tomatoes, rutabagas, cabbage and turnips.

After carefully examining a list of his daily foods, I observed, "Your diet seems short on protein and on at least three vitamins necessary to keep your thyroid working normally, particularly vitamin A."

That puzzled him.

"Something's wrong here, Doctor. I get plenty of vitamin A in carrots, sweet potatoes, spinach and tomatoes."

"That's not true. What you get in these vegetables is carotene, a precursor of vitamin A. An underactive thyroid gland cannot efficiently convert carotene to usable vitamin A. In addition, vegetables such as rutabagas, cabbage and turnips, eaten daily, suppress thyroid function even more."

That was just the surface aspect of Mark's thyroid deficiency. I pointed out that he lacked vitamins B2, B6 and B12, the former two further reducing his thyroid gland function. He rejected the idea of eating liver, which would have satisfied requirements for the B vitamins, so I recommended almonds, milk, wheat germ and brewer's yeast for vitamin B2; bananas, barley, wheat bran, wheat germ and brewer's yeast for vitamin B6 and, inasmuch as he wouldn't eat meat, the best other sources of vitamin B12—eggs, American and Swiss cheese and two kinds of fish, haddock and sole. I also put Mark on a grain of natural thyroid until the new diet could return his thyroid function to normal. Several months later this happened, and he is healthy again.

Although Mark's case was quite straightforward, that of Kathleen, a girl in her early teens, had mystified several other doctors and now challenged me. Once rather plump, ridiculed by schoolmates, she had opted for vegetarianism, despite parental objection, and had shed thirty-four pounds. Now she suffered from daily diarrhea, extreme sluggishness, and a seeming wasting away of muscles. She wore sunglasses even in my office.

"Is the light too bright?" I asked.

"Yes."

"Do you have any other eye problems?"

"It's a little hard for me to see at night," she replied.

"On a vegetarian diet, unless you work at it, it is difficult to take in enough protein—and enough of certain vitamins—to sustain you."

"My parents make me take a protein supplement twice every day," she responded.

That stopped me for an instant. However, her case triggered recall of a fascinating study done some years ago in India. Mass suffering from the protein deficiency disease kwashiorkor by tens of thousands of children prompted an American medical relief team to fly in to correct the situation. In kwashiorkor, the most prominent symptoms are wasting tissues, physical and mental sluggishness, swollen bellies, eye ailments—sometimes blindness—and even mental retardation. Immediately, the medical team fed the children a good grade of protein—powdered skim milk—expecting a reversal within weeks. Nothing beneficial happened, however, and they were baffled. Weeks ran into months, and the children grew steadily worse.

A second medical team flew in to help—doctors expert in eye ailments. Noting the myriad eye problems, they added vitamin A—a vitamin essential to good health of eyes—to the protein-enriched diet. Eye ailments began clearing up, and the children recovered from symptoms of protein deficiency. These doctors then ran painstaking tests and evaluated results, concluding that vitamin A must accompany protein to make it available to the body.

Kwashiorkor is a common disease in countries like India and parts of Africa and South America, where poverty prevents millions from eating enough protein and vitamin-A-rich foods such as meats and milk. Now how could a teenage girl in California show some of the symptoms of kwashiorkor? Apparently by following a diet not too different from those of kwashiorkor victims. I told my patient what had happened to the children in India, got her agreement to add milk products and eggs to her diet, gave her a good vitamin A supplement, vitamin B-complex and half a grain of thyroid to compensate for a malnourished thyroid gland. She did an amazing about-face. Today, she is a beautiful, slim, healthy young woman.

You may conclude from these cases that I do not favor a strict vegetarian diet; that is correct. Unless one is an experienced biochemist or nutritionist and knows the pedigrees of vegetables and fruit—that is, how they are grown, where, and with what kinds of fertilizers—it is difficult to secure enough protein and B vitamins.

Many years ago, Dr. William J. Albrecht of the University of Missouri investigated protein and vitamin content of commercially available vegetables and found that their food values had declined steadily because growers did not replace all the elements which the plants remove from the soil. Numerous more recent studies have shown the same alarming trend. Furthermore, vegetables and fruits contain only a negligible amount of vitamin B12. Most of us require just an infinitesimal amount of vitamin B12 daily—one microgram (one-millionth of a gram). If we don't get that much, however, we run the risk of pernicious anemia and possibly death. If my patients insist on strict vegetarianism, I tell them to proceed at their own peril, urging them to add milk, other dairy products and eggs as dietary insurance.

Not long ago I ran across a chilling item in the nationally syndicated newspaper column of Dr. Lawrence Power that demonstrates the hazards of uncompromising vegetarianism better than I can. Dr. Power cited a hospital report on twenty-five infants born in a religious community which adheres to a strict vegetarian diet. Twenty-five deathly ill babies were rushed to the hospital. Three were dead on arrival. Five more died short hours after admittance, all from malnutrition. The remaining seventeen—severely malnourished—were returned to good health by more complete nutrition. Upon entry into the hospital, the surviving infants had enteritis, pneumonia and anemia. Nine had acute rickets. The remainder showed involuntary muscle twitching.

I see too many risks in the Spartan vegetarian diet. Most vegetarians are opposed to eating red meat, but I see no reason why they can't include poultry and fish in their diets, or at least dairy products and eggs. (More about the value of eggs in the chapter on the heart.) The great peril of the strict vegetarian diet is suppression of the protective and life-giving thyroid function by minimizing the intake of essential vitamins.

In one of the most comprehensive published surveys of the effects of nutritional substances on thyroid health and function, Isobel Jennings of the University College, University of Cambridge, England, says in her biochemistry classic, *Vitamins in Endocrine Metabolism*, that carotene, the vitamin A precursor, is not easily translated into vitamin A.[1] Vitamin A is far better absorbed than carotene from vegetable sources, which is probably converted to vitamin A in the liver.

The malnutrition in the case of the babies mentioned earlier probably came about because infants (as well as adults with gastroenteritis) have a much reduced capacity for converting carotene to vitamin A. In hypothyroids and diabetics, this ability is nearly completely blocked. Without enough vitamin A, the infants could not make their limited protein supply available to their bodies.[2]

Just how do certain vitamin deficiencies affect the thyroid gland and its function? Studies cited by Isobel Jennings show that when animals are short-changed on vitamin A, their ability to produce thyroid-stimulating hormone (TSH) is limited. Vitamin A-deficient cattle and sheep show degeneration of pituitary gland basophils, the cells where TSH is synthesized.[3]

In the world of glands, the pituitary is king; it controls the structure and output of the thyroid gland by means of TSH and makes sure that there is enough thyroid hormone circulating in the blood to service the living cells. When this level has been reached, thyroid hormone (TH) shuts off production of TSH and inhibits the release of added TH. Vitamin A deficiency also influences the thyroid gland directly in two ways. The rate at which this gland can take up its major nutrient, iodine, is reduced, along with the amount of TH secreted.

A Danish researcher, B. Palludan, found that after two weeks of severe vitamin A deficiency, thyroid secretion of pigs was reduced by 40 to 50 percent. In other experiments, when thyroid glands were removed from rabbits, they developed bulging eyes, a condition called xerophthalmia. Administration of vitamin A corrected the eye disorder; carotene did not. Researchers have concluded that without a functioning thyroid—or adequate supplementation—vitamin A can be metabolized, but carotene cannot.

Like vitamin A, vitamin B2 (riboflavin) exerts a powerful influence on how well or how poorly the thyroid gland works. Animal experiments reveal that in a vitamin B2 shortage, function of the ovaries or testes is often depressed, and that changes occur in all glands—particularly in the thyroid and adrenals—which fail to secrete their hormones.[4]

Another powerful member of the vitamin B family, B3 (niacin), helps assure the good health of your thyroid and other glands. All living cells require niacin, since it assists in respiration and in the metabolism of carbohydrates, proteins and fats.[5] This vitamin is essential for keeping your cells—including those of your endocrine glands—in efficient working order.

A thyroid gland starved of vitamin B6 (pyridoxine) cannot

utilize its iodine raw material efficiently in the making of hormones that are a matter of life or death to us. Physiologists are not sure if this action is directly on the thyroid or on the pituitary gland, in which it may block the synthesis and release of TSH.[6]

Unless we feed the thyroid gland properly, we can't efficiently absorb another critical vitamin, B12 (cyanocobalamin). In laboratory tests, rats without thyroid glands could not absorb vitamin B12 at all.[7]

Earlier we mentioned that acute vitamin B12 deficiency could bring on death from pernicious anemia. Other serious symptoms are mental illness, various neurological disorders, neuralgia, neuritis and bursitis. This vitamin is one of the most temperamental of the B family. It can't be manufactured in our intestines and therefore must be ingested in foods or supplements. Some of us are not well enough supplied with what is called "the intrinsic factor," which makes it possible to absorb vitamin B12. Subnormal thyroid function is undoubtedly a little-known reason why many of us cannot make the best use of the vitamin B12 in our diets.

Although I do administer vitamin B12 shots to patients desperately low in this nutrient, I prefer to make certain that their thyroid is normal to assure proper absorption. Then, for non-vegetarians, I recommend the richest sources of B12: beef liver, beef kidney and beef round. Fortunately, many good vitamin B12 supplements are sold in nutrition stores. Hypothyroids usually show dramatic uptake of vitamin B12 once their blood levels of thyroid hormone are raised with natural desiccated thyroid supplement.

The thyroid gland is also hypersensitive to too little vitamin C (ascorbic acid) in the daily diet. When guinea pigs, which, unlike most of the lower animals, cannot synthesize ascorbic acid from other food substances, were made deficient in this vitamin, capillaries in the thyroid gland began bleeding, a condition which became even worse in acute scurvy. Additionally, in long-standing vitamin C deficiency, normal cells of the thyroid gland multiply at an abnormal rate—a condition called hyperplasia—and secrete too much hormone, as if the governing influence of the pituitary gland had been nullified. Once the guinea pigs were well supplied with vitamin C, all three negative conditions disappeared.

As is the case with depletion of ascorbic acid, experimental animals (rabbits) deficient in vitamin E showed unnaturally rapid multiplication of normal thyroid gland cells, as well as too little TSH synthesized by the pituitary gland.[8] Rats demonstrated the same basic response to deficiency of vitamin E, and, in addition, they transmitted hyperplasia to litters born to them. Most of the young failed to survive.[9]

A sense of horror comes over me when I think of the true significance of the last two experiments mentioned, namely, that a shortage of vitamins C and E brings about a condition which appears to be hyperthyroidism—over-production of thyroid hormone and a racing of the metabolic motor. What appalls me is that, from the turn of the century until the late 1950s, it was standard surgical procedure to remove the thyroid gland that was over- or under-productive. A great number of such operations might have been avoided merely by compensating for certain vitamin deficiencies.

To sum it all up, it is possible in many instances to correct unbalanced thyroid hormone production—too much or too little— merely by compensating for certain vitamin deficiencies. *Some cases of hypothyroidism can be successfully treated even without taking thyroid supplements.* Although most medical doctors are not noted for knowledge of nutrition, they should have at least basic information in this field so that they can treat patients correctly.

Some facts of life about nutrition and the thyroid have been known for the past twenty or thirty years. Yet they have never seen print in anything but medical publications, and there only rarely. One of this book's missions is to fill in the broad knowledge gap—to make you and your doctor aware that how and what you eat may be slowing down or speeding up your thyroid or even injuring it.

Individuals who have been proved to be hyperthyroid usually have part of their thyroid gland removed by surgery or by radiation. Some, however, are given chemicals such as thiouracil or thiourea to counteract over-production of hormone. Doctors who are not nutrition-oriented don't always realize that thiouracil and thiourea are thyroid antagonists, as Isobel Jennings points out. These drugs prevent conversion of carotene into usable vitamin A. Therefore, strict vegetarians suffer.[10] If the patient fails to take preformed vitamin A—not the carotene—he or she soon depletes vitamin A stores in the liver and kidneys. Then, because dietary protein cannot be used, the patient slowly declines into malnourishment. However, Isobel Jennings indicates that if the doctor prescribes thyroid supplementation to overcome the vitamin antagonists, carotene can be converted into vitamin A and assimilated, making protein absorption possible once more.

The overactive thyroid gland of the hyperthyroid individual has a hunger for vitamin B1 (thiamine), using much and excreting much. Therefore, a high intake of this vitamin is necessary.[11] Likewise, demand for vitamin B6 (pyridoxine) is high in hyperthyroidism and also when protein intake is generous. Depletion of this vitamin in hyperthyroidism is sometimes so great that only daily injection can prevent a common ailment, muscle weakness.[12] Other vitamins, too, are drawn upon heavily in hyperthyroidism, particularly vitamin C, which is literally drained from the tissues.[13] Some experimenters have found that the taking of vitamin D by hyperthyroids counteracts the usual rapid excretion of calcium, and the blood level of calcium returns to normal.[14] Higher intake of vitamin E is often needed as well to counteract the great amounts depleted from the system by this condition.[15]

Hyperthyroidism stimulates the metabolism of essential fatty acids (EFA), which the thyroid gland requires to function normally. Rats deprived of EFA become hyperactive with excessive thyroid hormone production. Experimenters do not yet know why this happens.[16]

A deficiency of EFA and vitamins is not the only cause of an unbalanced thyroid. Certain drugs and chemicals can suppress it as well. In a number of studies, sulfa drugs and antidiabetic agents interfered with the formation of thyroid hormones by inhibiting iodine uptake. It has been shown that prednisone should be used judiciously in known or suspected hypothyroidism, because, in pharmacologic doses, it indirectly worsens already abnormal thyroid function. So does estrogen in pharmacologic doses, an important consideration for women on birth control pills.

Heavy smokers should be aware that cigarette smoke contains thyocyanide, a fairly strong thyroid gland inhibitor. And since 1854, it has been known that fluoride is one of the most potent inhibitors of thyroid function, particularly where there is a low-to-deficient iodine concentration. Those who drink regularly from a fluoridated water supply and show a low temperature on the Barnes Basal Temperature Test may not be permanently hypothyroid. They may be experiencing thyroid suppression—a very good reason to use pure, bottled water.

This chapter will have done its job if it makes you aware that your diet, the water you drink and the medicines you take can cause your thyroid to behave abnormally. Now you have a new basis for examining your lifestyle in relation to your thyroid and, if necessary, for making positive changes. However, the place to start is with the Barnes Basal Temperature Test.

4

BODY HEAT

D r. Barnes's breakthrough research in hypothyroidism was
due in large part to his observations that patients with
thyroid deficiency were frequently cold even when people
in the same room were comfortable. Their cold hands and feet
created problems in social situations and in many instances
severely hampered their ability to have a harmonious sex life.

In addition, Dr. Barnes found that low body temperature inhibits the ability of these patients' bone marrow to produce both
red and white blood cells properly. Red blood cells are responsible for transporting oxygen to the rest of the body for food
metabolism, energy and heat. Red blood cell disturbances lead
to lower metabolic activity and still lower temperatures. Ability
of the marrow to produce white blood cells—soldiers of the

33

immune system army—is reduced, too, making hypothyroids vulnerable to repeated colds, flu, sinusitis, sore throat, pneumonia and other respiratory ailments.

While a physiology instructor at the University of Chicago many years ago, Dr. Barnes witnessed a dramatic demonstration that normal body temperature is essential to the production of sufficient blood cells. A Ph.D. candidate was puzzled as to why red and white blood cells were being formed only in the bone marrow of certain bones—the ribs, spine, pelvis and long bones nearest the body. "He suspected that it was a matter of temperature, body organs being warmer than the extremities (the arms and legs)," explains Dr. Barnes.

"To test this hypothesis, he devised a special needle in whose hollow he inserted a small, thin thermometer to check bone marrow temperature in a white rat. He found only yellow, non-bloodmaking marrow in the rat's long tail, whose temperature, indeed, was lower than that of the blood-producing backbone.

"Then he curved the rat's tail, made a small incision in the animal's belly, temporarily inserting and suturing the tail there. Soon the marrow in the tip of the tail, now warmed by the body, was transformed into blood-producing red marrow, while the marrow of the bony structure of the tail's curve remained yellow and unable to make blood cells."

Years later in his medical practice, this graphic demonstration helped Dr. Barnes understand why anemic women often remain dragged out, pale and depressed, even after having been administered extra iron. Several hundred sickly patients regained a new, fuller life when he gave them thyroid supplementation, which raised their temperature and increased their body's ability to produce blood cells, particularly red corpuscles.

Supplemental iron therapy is usually only temporarily useful in the treatment of hypothyroid anemia, because it treats the symptoms, rather than the cause, which is well taken care of by thyroid hormone therapy. Foods rich in iron—liver, fish, fowl, meats, fruit, green vegetables, raisins and brown rice—are of limited value in a person whose anemia is caused by a hypothyroid condition.

At best, the body absorbs little more than 10 percent of available iron. Vitamin C (ascorbic acid) greatly aids the absorption of iron from the digestive tract. Research done by Drs. Paul R.

McCurdy of Georgetown University School of Medicine and Raymond J. Dern of Loyola University Stritch School of Medicine revealed that between 200 and 500 mg of ascorbic acid made it possible for the body to absorb twice as much iron (ferrous sulphate, 15 to 120 mg) as without this vitamin.[1] An accompanying dose of 500 mg of vitamin C resulted in a much higher absorption of iron from the gut than when smaller doses of this vitamin were given. A Swedish study, in fact, revealed that the United States government's recommended daily allowance (RDA) of 60 mg of vitamin C will do nothing to help absorb iron.[2]

Once absorbed, iron is constantly recycled by the body to manufacture new red blood cells from worn-out ones. Women, however, lose iron with their menstrual flow, and must therefore replace it in their diet. After absorption, iron must be assimilated by the cells in order to manufacture the hemoglobin necessary to carry oxygen throughout the body. To enable this to happen, another essential mineral, copper—found in liver, other organ meats, bone meal, legumes, molasses, nuts, raisins and seafood—must be present.[3] If, as is often the case, copper is in short supply, the blood's oxygen-carrying efficiency may be sharply diminished.

Hypothyroidism may reduce the uptake of copper from the gastrointestinal tract. In addition, a decreased body temperature, common to an underactive thyroid, can cause brain wave changes which may be misinterpreted by a clinician as neurological damage, but which will in most instances be entirely reversible when thyroid therapy is instituted.

Slower reaction time is caused by lowered body temperature, as illustrated by polar explorers subjected to extreme cold who develop hypothermia. Anyone who is hypothyroid may have similar complaints.

Emanuel Donchin, a psychologist, and Noel K. Marshall, an electrophysicist, both of the Cognitive Psychophysiology Laboratory at the University of Illinois, discovered, not long ago, that seemingly small daily changes in body temperature—one or two degrees below normal—reduce certain brain responses in test subjects.[4] Their findings showed that even slightly depressed body temperatures slow down our movements and our higher thought processes. Although we may not be aware of it, our brains respond more slowly to sound.

Brain wave peaks have a readily recognizable pattern. Nerve damage in the brain is a good possibility if wave peaks either don't appear or come later than they should. In hypothermia, the brain wave peaks are markedly delayed. Yet when the temperatures of these subjects are normalized, the brain waves speed up and become normal.

Donchin and Marshall caution doctors diagnosing such cases to consider body temperature of patients before concluding that they have irreversible brain damage. This recommendation was based on their experiments with fifteen test subjects. They discovered that even small temperature changes caused changes in their test subjects. The efficiency of sensory processing and coordination dropped with subnormal temperatures and rose when temperatures reached normal.

These scientists relate their findings to those of G. A. Kerkhof and his colleagues at the University of Leiden (Netherlands), who discovered that body temperatures actually do influence the brain in a manner that correlates with how subjects rate their performance of various tasks.[5]

Sometimes we put ourselves into categories—as "morning" or "evening" people—according to our work efficiency. Kerkhof discovered that temperatures were normal at peak performance times and lower than normal at other times. Not only was execution better at peak times, but subjects could also concentrate longer when working.

Experiments by Kerkhof and Donchin and Marshall offer laboratory proof of the handicaps of those individuals with a chronically low temperature, as in hypothyroidism. Frequently hypothyroids register temperatures from one to two and a half degrees below normal, as I have observed many times in my practice.

Now we can better understand why persons with extremely low thyroid function—and correspondingly low temperatures— show some of the following symptoms: slow-motion response, thick-tongued speech, poor coordination, impaired memory and a slowing of mental activity.

If, indeed, 40 percent of the American population suffers from hypothyroidism, an incredible amount of mental and physical potential is being lost needlessly, because no condition can be more readily and inexpensively treated than hypothyroidism. Yet none is more frequently untreated and, even worse, unsuspected. Unless this condition is corrected, the thyroid gland, in partnership with the adrenal glands, cannot properly operate the body's heat-regulating system.[6] That is why so many hypothyroids are cold when everybody else in the room is warm.

Not only do these glands regulate body heat for everyday living, they raise the body's temperature in disease states to produce a fever, which protects us from infection. Ever since the first thermometer was invented, there has been a difference of opinion about fever. Is it a friend or an enemy? The only point doctors have agreed on in the past hundred years is that fever is a sign of illness.

In the early twentieth century, the eminent physician Sir William Osler labeled fever as one of the three great scourges of mankind, the other two being famine and war: "By far the greatest, by far the most terrible is fever," he concluded.[7] Even the eminent can be wrong. However, in 1960, two scientists, I. L. Bennett, Jr., and A. Nicastri, did a thorough review of medical literature and, although not as extreme in their judgment as Sir William, they found no convincing evidence that fever benefits us in our continual warfare with microbes.[8]

Then researcher M. J. Kluger and his associates blasted this opinion with a stunning discovery on infected lizards. Lizards do not have a built-in fever-generating system such as ours and must find fever-inducing sources on the outside.[9] The Kluger team learned that sick lizards have an instinct which makes them seek hot environments in order to raise their body temperatures to fever level when they are sick. Infected fish, too, swim to warmer water to raise their temperatures and combat illness.

Various experimenters have discovered that fever encourages quick inflammation in the immediate area of an infection and keeps it from spreading. Apparently fever is triggered in the brain first by a hormone-like substance from macrophages, immune system cells that attack invading germs. Then the thyroid gland and adrenal glands work together to speed up metabolism to produce extreme heat.

Experiments by G. W. Duff and S. K. Durum showed that at two degrees centigrade of fever, certain immune system defenders—T-cells and antibodies—increased by 2000 percent over their number at normal body temperature.[10] Similar findings were reported by another research team. Antibody production in the spleen cells has been found to increase dramatically during a fever. Scientists have concluded that the hormone-like substances, called interleukin-1, set off body defense cells to fight infection and also send the brain signals to increase body temperature to provide an ideal climate for the multiplication of defense cells. Many physiologists believe that human beings are equipped with a temperature regulation system which puts a ceiling on fever at approximately 41.11 degrees centigrade (106 degrees Fahrenheit). In heat stroke and malignant hyperthermia, temperature breaks through to killing levels.

How is fever controlled? Scientists are not sure. Some believe that fever lingers as long as the infection lasts and recedes when there is no longer need for it.

If fever increases our ability to fight diseases, do subnormal temperatures make us more susceptible to them? Very likely. Hypothyroidism and its accompanying subnormal temperatures are stresses which lower the body's innate ability to fight off infection.

We are always under attack by infectious agents—bacteria and viruses. Countless invisible enemies mass on the skin, in the mouth and throat and in the intestinal tract. Yet that is only half the bulletin from the war zones. Our built-in resistance, our own defense network, is the other half. If we keep our resistance high enough, the enemy cannot win the battle. He is neutralized until some stress weakens us and permits him to multiply and grow stronger.

Low thyroid function is far from the only stress that invites attack. Devastating emotional shock, long exposure to extreme heat or cold, physical exertion, inferior nutrition, insufficient sleep are other common causes of weakened resistance. But, hypothyroidism is definitely a major stress. Subnormal body temperature and too little thyroid hormone can reduce the strength and resistance of every cell, including the billions involved in the immune system. One of the most common results of hypothyroidism which I see daily in my office is recurrent colds, throat and nose infections and other respiratory ailments.

Between sniffles and a hacking cough, a patient named Beverly let out all her frustration on the first visit to my office.

"Dr. Langer, I feel as if the common cold was invented exclusively for me. I'm sick at least four times a year—winter, spring, summer and fall. I've had every respiratory ailment through the alphabet from A to Z."

Beverly's sardonic humor fascinated me, because it seemed too vigorous in contrast with her many symptoms typical of hypothyroidism: low energy, cold extremities, an assortment of respiratory ailments, tight, mask-like facial skin and a more than plump figure.

A Barnes Basal Temperature reading of 96.4 degrees confirmed my suspicion. I started Beverly on a grain of natural thyroid, two tablespoons of brewer's yeast (taken an hour before breakfast and lunch in grapefruit juice to prevent flatulence) and 10,000 units of vitamin A, plus 3000 milligrams of vitamin C daily. Several weeks later, she returned, looking great, weighing six pounds less, all smiles and no sniffles.

"This treatment seems to have broken my monopoly on respiratory ailments," she proudly announced.

And she was right.

Another new patient, whom I'll call Diane, had a similar problem but one with sad social overtones. A natural auburn-haired woman in her mid-thirties, she would have been striking, except for many symptoms of respiratory problems—a slightly swollen, reddish nose, watery green eyes and a nervous habit of continually clearing her throat.

"Doctor, I simply can't shake this cold, no matter what cold remedies I take." She covered a sneeze with Kleenex. "I go through a big box of Kleenex every other day. I'm desperate. I don't know what to do."

Fortunately, I did. I had never seen a naturally red-haired patient who was not at least slightly hypothyroid. Comparing notes with other hypothyroid-aware doctors, including Dr. Barnes, I found corroboration. An auburn-haired person who is not hypothyroid is a rare bird. No one has been able to explain why.

In any event, Diane's condition depressed her, because, with her frequent sneezing, nose-blowing, throat-clearing and headaches, men avoided her.

"Nobody wants me and my cold," she said. "I'm like Typhoid Mary." Tears of frustration began rolling down her cheeks.

Diane had so many obvious symptoms of hypothyroidism that

I didn't delay giving her a grain of natural thyroid even before getting a report on her temperature, which, it turned out, was two degrees subnormal. Nothing dramatic happened for three weeks. Then Diane phoned to say the mucus was clearing from her head. "I'm beginning to feel like a human being." After three months, she was a total human being, and an extremely beautiful one. The headaches and respiratory ailments had all disappeared. She hadn't had any symptoms of a cold for weeks and felt great.

"You probably don't recognize me without a wad of Kleenex in my hand," she said during her last office visit, when she promised to stay on thyroid supplementation for the rest of her life. I haven't seen Diane for years. I know I would have if she weren't feeling well. What a pleasure to lose a patient to good health!

Diane's case is not uncommon. Often I have found unyielding colds and related respiratory ailments interfering with patients' love lives. The same goes for headaches, a frequent symptom of hypothyroidism. Many headaches in the bedroom are not just bedroom headaches. They are real ones. I have helped hundreds of patients get rid of them without aspirin.

Every part of the body suffers when insufficient thyroid hormones are available, including the skin and even the erogenous zones. A poor complexion is often a revealing sign of hypothyroidism, although far less dependable than subnormal basal temperature. Sophisticated electronic measuring devices have shown that in extreme cases of low thyroid function, the skin may be deprived of 75 to 80 percent of its normal blood supply, severely reducing the amount of nourishment delivered to the cells and delaying the removal of harmful waste products.[11] All sorts of strange, embarrassing skin conditions can result, disorders damaging to social and sexual acceptance: blackheads, whiteheads, pimples, boils, carbuncles, acne, eczema, icthyosis (fish skin) and psoriasis, among others. Thyroid therapy brings about almost unbelievable improvement, often complete disappearance of these conditions, because circulation has been stepped up. Further, the sensitivity of erogenous zones to touch and friction is heightened, making sex more enjoyable. Conditions which make sex less enjoyable—fatigue, headaches, respiratory ailments and being physically cold—tend to diminish or vanish with thyroid supplementation.

To the hypothyroid with low body heat and a string of related physical problems, survival is higher on the priority list than love-making. But in time, thyroid supplements may be able to effect a remarkable change in priorities!

5

THYROID AND SEX—
FOR WOMEN

*O*ut of the memorable Broadway musical *Flower Drum Song* came an exuberant song, "I Enjoy Being a Girl," which unfortunately does not express the sentiments of many women just before and during the menstrual period. Ever since Eve, women have agonized each month, losing valuable time from work, education, social activities, recreation and sports, while the male-dominated medical professssion had done little or nothing to help.

Likewise, ever since the bedroom went public in the sexual revolution, women—and men—have developed inferiority feelings about their contributions to love-making, comparing them to survey results and fictional standards. I know this from my own practice in preventive medicine and from discussions with numerous physicians, including gynecologists.

Few women *or* men know that a properly functioning or supplemented thyroid gland can bring new excitement to their sexuality. Even fewer know that the Pill, an effective birth control method, can cause severe bodily damage in hypothyroidism.

In this chapter I will discuss menstrual disorders, sexual problems, sexual enjoyment and birth control as they relate to proper thyroid function.

To help women cope with menstrual problems, I have administered, although unwillingly, pain-killers, aspirin, relaxants and tranquilizers. These are alien chemical substances which can be harmful, and therefore I prefer to use natural means. By administering desiccated thyroid, I have seen the correction or at least the lessening of such menstrual disorders as inordinate pain, irregularity, too copious flow or premature or delayed menses.

Dr. Broda Barnes has managed almost two thousand such cases successfully by this method and has given me access to his findings. He told me that he almost felt like shouting "Eureka!" when he first found thyroid supplementation to be helpful for these problems.

"I experienced the exultation of a pioneer until medical history revealed that, as early as 1899, Dr. Eugene Hertoghe, of Antwerp, Belgium, had discovered that many female problems result from mild to acute thyroid deficiency," he admitted. "He cured hundreds of women with thyroid supplements. Incidentally, his grandson is achieving the same success today, as I learned not long ago while lecturing on thyroid to a group of physicians in Belgium." The Hertoghe method spread to the United States in the early 1900s, bringing welcome relief to tens of thousands of women.

Early medical textbooks and journal articles mentioned the effectiveness of thyroid supplementation in problems peculiar to women. In the 1950 Curtis-Huffman *Textbook of Gynecology*, the authors wrote that even medical conservatives accept that thyroid substance has definite value.[1] It is helpful in promoting conception, in stopping functional uterine bleeding from various causes, in improving gynecological disturbances in many patients with a low metabolic rate, in correcting delayed onset of menstruation in adolescents and, most especially, in adjusting disorders of menstrual flow.

Taylor's *Essentials of Gynecology*, published in 1969, states that in myxedema (acutely subnormal thyroid function) pre-menopausal patients may show menstrual excesses and this condition may be corrected with thyroid extract.[2] Dr. Taylor relates that one researcher (Lerman) discovered that the hypothyroid patient has a loss of normal follicle-stimulating hormone (the substance which spurs growth of cells surrounding the eggs in the ovaries) preceding menopause. In patients past menopause, Lerman found that follicle-stimulating hormone levels were lower than in normal patients of the same age. He also learned that treatment of hypothyroidism with thyroid hormones was accompanied by a rise in follicle-stimulating hormone.

"Occasionally, amenorrhea [interruption of normal menstrual periods] will be a complication of hypothyroidism," wrote Dr. Taylor. "With correction of the hypothyroidism, regular menstrual cycles will follow."

In a study of fatigued hypothyroid women with menstrual disorders, Mayo Clinic researchers administered thyroid hormone to bring their metabolism to normal range.[3] Numerous gynecological conditions improved: amenorrhea improved in 72 percent of the women; aligomenorrhea (deficient menstruation) in 55 percent and menorrhagia (excessive blood flow) in 73 percent. A bonus value was an improvement in the health of 75 percent of the women, including higher energy levels.

A recent experiment reported in the *International Journal of Gynecological Obstetrics* illustrates that just one component of the thyroid hormone, thyroxin, helps restore menstruation in women with low-normal thyroid function. Regular menstrual cycles were restored in ten of seventeen test subjects.[4] An article published in another international journal, *Problems of Endokrinology*, revealed that in a study of twenty-three infertile female hypothyroids with amenorrhea and lactorrhea, most were returned to normal by thyroid therapy.[5]

A third article, this one in the *Journal of Endocrinology*, established a "distinct relationship between thyroid function and that of the ovary ..." in a bird experiment.[6]

Thyroid hormones, too, are essential to the proper development of the breast, as shown by animal experiments. They help to regulate the growth and development of the mammary gland. By decreasing the levels of thyroid hormone in the blood, researchers were able to retard the growth of key parts of the breast.[7]

Although hypothyroidism contributes to many kinds of female problems, the most widespread in my practice are menstrual, even though I am not a gynecologist. This is also true for Dr. Barnes, who scanned his office files on 2,051 adult female patients with a complete menstrual history and was amazed to find that 1,980 of them (80 percent) had some kind of female problem. Of these, 1,590 had had menstrual cramps; 883 had had irregular periods, usually accompanied by cramps; and the remainder had undergone occasional flooding or had had an early or late onset of menstruation.

Those with menstrual distress experienced moderate to severe pain (a day or two of school or work lost each month), although some patients endured more excruciating pain than often accompanies having a baby, with no baby to show for it.

Individuals whose menstrual periods started later than the average age of twelve numbered 438. The oldest was eighteen. Those whose periods started too early numbered 260, the youngest being a five-year-old who also developed mature breasts and pubic hair. Immediately recognized as hypothyroid, she was treated with low-potency natural desiccated thyroid and in a month menstruation stopped, the breasts started regressing and pubic hair disappeared until puberty.

In most of Dr. Barnes's cases—and in mine, as well—painful menstruation, irregularity, too copious flow and premature or delayed menses normalized with administration of thyroid supplementation. The type of uterine bleeding brought about by low thyroid function runs to opposite extremes—excessive flow to sparse flow. A word of caution: abnormal blood flow may be a sign of uterine cancer, so it makes sense to be checked by a gynecologist.

If thyroid function is normal and menstrual irregularities continue, certain vitamin deficiencies may be the cause. A lack of vitamin B12 or folic acid has been found to bring on irregularity, sparse flow or no flow, conditions which are corrected when the missing vitamins are supplied.

A heavy menstrual flow for three or four days has often been corrected if the patient takes 600 international units of vitamin E daily for thirty days. Sometimes a damaged liver—which cannot inactivate hormones which govern menstruation—may cause a too-copious flow. Liver damage can result from alcoholism, a diet high in sugar or other refined carbohydrates or saturated fats, or from deficiencies of calcium, magnesium or protein (particularly the amino acids cystine and methionine) or vitamins A and C, which, with choline, are protectors of the liver.

Like menstrual problems, sexual dysfunction (once called frigidity, an insensitive, finger-pointing word) can arise from one or more factors: fatigue, illness, dyspareunia (pain during the sexual act), guilt feelings, self-consciousness, and emotional tension with one's mate, to name some of the common ones. A spectrum of supercharged emotional problems can contribute, too: indelicate treatment in the first sexual encounter, rape, a hangover from childhood conditioning to taboos of sex, a lingering attachment to a parent. Some can be so traumatic and unyielding that they need psychological or psychiatric treatment. Physical problems, some common, some not so common, can contribute, too: irritation or infection of the vulva or vagina, the injured remainder of the hymen, the bruised tissue from abortion or crudely executed surgery in the mouth of the vagina to aid delivery in difficult childbirth.

Even seemingly insignificant factors can bring on discomfort in intercourse. A patient with a sinus infection complained of secreting too little lubrication for enjoyable sex. Inasmuch as antihistamines are drying agents, I told her to stop taking them, cleared up her sinus infection with penicillin, and soon she was again forming ample lubrication.

Both physical and emotional obstacles to sexual enjoyment—fatigue, vague illnesses and even childhood conditioning against sex—are often overcome by thyroid supplementation.

A patient we'll call Linda told me bitterly, "I don't feel a thing during love-making."

She showed a low score of 96.8 degrees on the Barnes Basal Temperature Test. Clinical symptoms and her medical history told me plainly that she was hypothyroid, and I prescribed the natural desiccated thyroid supplement.

"Thyroid? How can that possibly help?" she asked incredulously.

I explained that the electrocardiogram (EKG) of hypothyroid

individuals shows reduced nerve stimulation of the heart muscle, causing blood to be pumped in lesser quantities and less forcefully. Reduced nerve conduction influences not only the heart but many other parts of the body, often desensitizing the sex organs.

This patient's response to thyroid supplementation was cheering: a temperature rise to normal and ecstatic reaction to lovemaking including, for the first time, sexual climax.

Another satisfying case was that of a young woman named Ardis.

"Doctor, I'm cold physically and sexually. I'm never spontaneous in bed," she confessed. "It's probably my puritanical upbringing. My husband wants to trade me in for a better model." She paused with a sigh. "Maybe I should be seeing a psychiatrist."

I shook my head. "No. You came to the right place."

The armpit test showed her to be markedly hypothyroid, so I prescribed a grain of thyroid daily. During her fourth visit, Ardis beamed:

"My hands, feet and the rest of me are warm now," she bubbled. "How I enjoyed sex last night! I wasn't at all self-conscious."

Thyroid supplementation has fanned many fires, banishing bedroom headaches and guilt feelings. Aside from its values in heightening sexual urge and the enjoyment of sex, thyroid therapy helps marriage become more productive. One authority told the Section of Obstetrics and Gynecology of the American Medical Association that 30 percent of sterile women with low thyroid function conceived while on thyroid supplements.[8]

Before thyroid treatment was pushed into the background by the plethora of drugs from the arsenal of the pharmaceutical industry, a gynecology textbook by Emil Novak, of Johns Hopkins Medical School, stated that, in hypothyroids, thyroid therapy will usually correct menstrual disorders, infertility and miscarriage.[9] In these times, however, less accent is put on sex for procreation. Most patients seem more interested in birth control, in finding the elusive, foolproof way of avoiding pregnancy. The Pill currently enjoys the greatest popularity, because of its effectiveness and convenience.

The Pill distributes its two major ingredients—estrogen and progestin (synthetic female hormone) throughout the body's cells, acting to prevent the ovaries from producing eggs. Among other things, it creates a hostile environment for pregnancy, thinning the endometrium (uterine lining) while decreasing its secretions.

I am unenthusiastic about the use of drugs which are not absolutely necessary, especially powerful ones with well-documented side effects, such as the Pill, which is contraindicated for women with asthma, cystic breast disease, a family history of breast cancer, diabetes, blood-clotting disorders, high blood pressure, heart, kidney and liver disease, exposure to DES before birth, elevated blood serum cholesterol or triglycerides; epilepsy, fibroid uterine tumors, gallbladder disease, menstrual abnormalities, migraine headaches and the habit of smoking.

In addition to women with these problems, I flatly refuse to prescribe the Pill for anyone older than thirty-five. The momentum of risk gains dizzy speed with each year after that age. I prescribe it only if would-be users are safeguarded against blood-clotting disorders by adequate thyroid function or by thyroid supplementation. Of more than 100 patients in my practice who took the Pill for less than five years, not one developed any of the wide range of common side effects: blood-clotting disorders, high blood pressure, strokes, heart attacks, migraine headaches, eye ailments and liver tumors, among others.

I have been well guided by a report which Dr. Barnes wrote for *Federation Proceedings* (a copy of which he gave me for my patients' benefit and for use in this book) called "Making the Pill Safer with Thyroid."[10] In it he states:

> The most serious complication from oral contraceptives has been a seven to tenfold increase in morbidity and mortality due to thromboembolic diseases reported in Great Britain. Another British report states that the Pill causes an elevation in low density lipoproteins, triglycerides and cholesterol levels in the serum.
>
> Since these changes are characteristic of abnormalities found in thyroid deficiencies, and since some cases of rapid coagulation are found in hypothyroidism, it would appear that a careful scrutiny of thyroid function should be made in all cases before initiating the Pill. The Basal Temperature has been found to be the most satisfactory test. If a woman has any symptoms of thyroid deficiency and/or a subnormal Basal Temperature, adequate thyroid therapy is maintained as long as she is taking the Pill.
>
> In my large general practice, no case of thrombophlebitis has

occurred, and few patients have complained of water retention. Thyroid is an excellent diuretic in hypothyroidism. A few cases have been seen in which thrombophlebitis developed under administration of the Pill from other physicians.

In each instance, evidence of thyroid deficiency has been present before the contraceptive was started. Thyroid prophylaxis for thromboses in those taking the Pill seems to be as effective as it is for the prevention of coronary disease.

On the heels of scare stories about the problems with oral contraceptives, many women are going to intrauterine devices (IUDs). However, various studies reveal that IUDs bring on an increased risk of pelvic inflammatory disease (PID), which can cause infertility. A survey by David W. Kaufman and coworkers at the Boston University School of Medicine uncovered some frightening facts. Of 460 women observed and questioned, all of whom used IUDs or another form of contraception, 150 had pelvic disease. IUD users run a nine times greater risk of developing PID than do women utilizing other birth control methods, the study disclosed. Results printed in the *Journal of the American Medical Association* showed the comparative risks, starting with the highest. Dalkon Shield users are 79 times more likely to acquire PID than non-IUD users. Those who utilized the Lippes Loop ran a 13 times greater risk than non-IUD users, and those fitted with copper IUDs had seven times the risk factor of non-users.[11]

Obviously, there are hazards in almost every form of birth control. However, if the ground rules are adhered to with the Pill, this method seems to have many advantages. Most birth control methods are not fair, in that they place the responsibility entirely on the woman. But now there is a way that men can share responsibility—not just by the obvious means of vasectomy, a surgical procedure which some males live to regret. This will be discussed in the next chapter.

6

THYROID AND SEX—
FOR MEN

I thought I had heard everything when a new patient, twenty-six-year-old Clayton, sole owner of a small manufacturing company, admitted to using the headache alibi when his wife wanted sex more often than he could deliver. In this liberated society, bedroom headaches are no longer the sole prerogative of women!

Already a workaholic, Clayton avoided embarrassment over the test of his maleness—"or lack of it," as he put it—by also taking refuge in long hours of work in his plant. As the story unfolded, the problem came into sharp focus. Within five years, Clayton had translated a patent into a thriving production firm through the usual entrepreneurial formula: a clear-cut goal—wishing to become a millionaire through his inventiveness—little capital and many long, grueling hours. To Clayton, the first one at the plant early each morning and the last to leave late at night, weekends were just two more weekdays. Obviously, he had not only worked at a sprint but could have made the *Guinness Book of World Records* for rapid eating. He bolted two-minute meals from the lunch wagon, gulped eleven cups of coffee daily and chomped endless glazed donuts, sweet rolls or cookies "to get me through the day and night."

Fear of bedroom failure and embarrassment compounded Clayton's intermittent impotency. Diagnosis? Emotional causes compounded by physical ones: exhaustion (never calculated to enhance sexuality), little sleep and relaxation, junk foods (as nourishing as wartime prison camp fare, which rendered many men temporarily incapable sexually) and subnormal thyroid function.

I advised Clayton to level with his wife—to tell her that he was under doctor's orders not to have sexual demands placed on him until his total recovery—and also to delegate tasks, to stop suicidal fourteen- to sixteen-hour workdays, to take weekends off, to get more sleep and to cut out junk foods. I told him to improve his diet by adding more protein, fresh vegetables and food supplements: brewer's yeast, desiccated liver and wheat germ, plus vitamins C, D and E, essential fatty acids (in the form of evening primrose oil) and the minerals selenium, calcium, magnesium and potassium. After finding that his basal temperature was 96.2 degrees, I put Clayton on a daily grain of natural thyroid. This regime turned him around in three months. Then the power of his sex drive overcame his self-consciousness and fear of failure, and he recovered completely.

Like Clayton, many men feel their masculinity being tested, even threatened, by the increased aggressiveness of women in initiating sex—a good reason for them to make sure that their thyroid function is normal and that they are in peak condition otherwise.

Aside from wanting to feel equal to sexual demands on them, male patients appear to be assuming more responsibility for birth control, as evidenced by a growing number of vasectomies. Because of the difficulty of reversing vasectomy, many men want to know if there is an effective means of contributing to birth control without surgery.

I tell them about something promising on the horizon. Not long ago, British medical researchers accidentally discovered an efficient birth-control product. While taking a heart medication called beta blockers, men complained to doctors that they couldn't make their wives pregnant. To investigate, researchers put a drop of the drug into vigorously swimming sperm. Within ten seconds, the sperm lay dead. After testing is done to determine if all men can use the drug safely, and after governmental approvals are secured, men may be able to assume responsibility for birth control.

As interesting as this subject is, most men are mainly preoccupied with making sure that their sexual ability meets or exceeds demand. This fact did not come to light immediately relative to a new patient of mine, a bright, thirty-one-year-old insurance salesman whom I'll call Jerry. His problem was irregular heartbeat.

I was perplexed. Jerry had no history of illness. The diet sheet he had filled out revealed no clue. My questions turned up nothing helpful except that occasionally he seemed hesitant, guarded. Obviously, he was holding out on me. Sometimes patients did that when asked about their sex lives.

"Look, Jerry, you came to me with a problem," I said bluntly. "You're not telling me things that could let me help you."

He flushed.

"Tell me, what have you been doing differently in the past month or so that might account for your problem?"

"I'm having trouble with my sex life," he admitted.

It turned out he was having a problem getting an erection. Sometimes it didn't stay hard for more than a few minutes. Once it softened on him during sexual intercourse, and he was humiliated.

"What did you do about it?" I asked.

"I began taking zinc. That's supposed to be the sexy mineral."

I agreed with him silently. The prostate gland and its secretions have a high content of zinc, as do the sperm cells. Potency and fertility disorders often yield to supplementation with zinc and its vitamin companion, B6. Zinc is essential in the formation and function of a number of sex hormones, including gonadotrophin, which excites and stimulates the sex glands of males and females. One medical paper had shown that without zinc, no gonadotrophin could be produced.

"Zinc certainly contributes importantly to sex drive, enjoyment and fulfillment," I told him.

"I felt I couldn't get enough zinc from my diet," he said. "I read in an article that zinc content of grains—corn, oats and wheat—has dropped 10 percent or more in recent years."

"True. Some studies show that zinc and other trace minerals are being taken out of the soil year after year and not returned. What is happening to farm land is similar to what is happening to money values through the invisible larceny of inflation."

"My zinc supplement helped me sexually to a degree," he went on.

"How much zinc are you taking daily?"

"Just a small amount, about 100 milligrams."

This remark upset me.

"*Just* 100 milligrams a day? Jerry, that's a lot. You can't take trace minerals in the liberal amounts that you can many vitamins."

Then I remembered a talk given by Jeffrey Bland, Ph.D., Professor of Nutritional Biochemistry at the University of Puget Sound. He and I, along with Dr. Barnes, had been speakers at a symposium for medical doctors in Texas on the subject of hypothyroidism. Dr. Bland had done some original research on zinc and copper and their relationship to low thyroid function and had studied the literature on this subject for many years. Something Dr. Bland had said told me what Jerry's trouble was. He had probably upset the natural ratio of zinc to copper in his body.

Quickly, I skimmed over Jerry's food chart to confirm my opinion.

"I don't find seafood on your chart."

"I don't eat it too often."

"How about organ meats—kidneys, brains, sweetbreads, liver?"

"Never."

"How about nuts?"

"Once in a while."

"Those are copper-containing foods. What I suspect is that you've disturbed your zinc-copper ratio. Many biochemists feel that we get all the copper we need from our foods and don't have to supplement. Therefore, if we increase our zinc intake as you have—and the ratio for most individuals is eight parts of zinc to one of copper—we throw off the relationship. You can't safely bring your copper level up with the very high intake of zinc, because you would be risking copper intoxication."

I told him that Dr. Bland had found that irregular heartbeats, premature beats and other EKG abnormalities were caused in animals by a diet deficient in copper and had been corrected by the addition of minute amounts of copper in their diet.[2] Dr. Bland had cited similar results in human test subjects.

I asked Jerry to reduce his zinc intake to no more than 30 to 40 mg daily and to add 4 mg of copper. Within two weeks his heart irregularity stopped. I found his thyroid function a bit low and added a grain of thyroid to his daily regimen.

Not long ago, Jerry told me, "My sex life is great again, and my heart is fine."

So many thanks that I get from patients should actually go to thyroid pioneers like Dr. Barnes and to unsung biochemical pioneers like Dr. Jeffrey Bland.

Copper and zinc are important trace minerals, vital in a number of bodily functions including the sexual. I remembered clearly that Dr. Bland had mentioned that the list of symptoms for zinc and copper deficiencies was almost identical to that for hypothyroidism. He had also said that trace minerals within human beings act as coenzymes. Enzymes are molecules which cause biochemical changes without being changed themselves. They cause carbohydrates to be split into simple sugars, fats to be broken into fatty acids and proteins into amino acids. There are, in addition, thousands of other enzymatic actions.

Some enzymes can't act on their own—metalo enzymes, for instance. They have to become bound to trace minerals such as zinc and copper to work. So if there is not enough zinc or copper or any other trace mineral to go around, certain enzymes can't become attached to them and do their proper job. Metalo enzymes work in the brain, the liver, the heart and every other body organ and tissue.

One kind of copper-containing molecule is necessary to oxidize iron and change it to a form acceptable in hemoglobin molecules—that which carries oxygen throughout the arterial system.

"There are many people in our population with an anemia that doesn't respond to iron supplementation," says Dr. Bland. "They are truly suffering from copper insufficiency."[3]

Without another kind of copper-containing enzyme, the skin could not accept pigmentation. One of the first signs of copper deficiency is called "subtle albinism," an extremely white skin, which tans poorly and sometimes develops white spots. Still another copper-containing enzyme concentrates heavily in the adrenal gland, which could not synthesize norepinephrine, one of its key hormones, without this enzyme.

Two more copper-dependent enzymes guard against body deterioration: superoxide dismutase (SOD), a compound well-known for protecting individual cells from attack by free radicals (chemicals which cause our bodies to age), and a metalo enzyme which forms elastin, one of the integral parts of the artery walls.

Likewise, five zinc-bound enzymes make life-or-death contributions. One of them controls the rate of protein synthesis, cell growth, cell repair, hair growth and white blood cell production. A second zinc-bound enzyme is an important part of the first step in metabolizing alcohol. A third zinc-containing enzyme contributes to the manufacture of retinaldehyde, a pigment which makes night vision possible. Still another one enables us to enjoy a full sense of smell and taste. Zinc-deficient people often lose the ability to smell, or objects give off a strange odor to them. The fifth zinc-attached enzyme helps to clear lactate from muscles and joints. In shortages of this trace element, muscle and joint pains are more acute.

On this subject, Dr. Bland mentioned a little-known fact based on an authoritative published paper which says that many symptoms of old age are really not the results of the aging process, but rather the results of malnutrition, including a deficiency of trace minerals.

These metalo enzymes create many symptoms similar to those of hypothyroidism, but do they in fact have a direct influence on thyroid function? They do in several ways. Before going into them, it might be well to mention again that the thyroid gland is activated, first, by thyroid-releasing hormone (TRH) from the hypothalamus gland by way of the pituitary gland, which gives off thyroid-stimulating hormone (TSH) to urge the thyroid into releasing its hormones into the bloodsteam.

According to Dr. Bland, "neurotransmitters in the brain and the TRH from the hypothalamus and the TSH from the pituitary are controlled by copper nutrition." How well the thyroid hormone thyroxin (T4) is metabolized in our trillions of cells depends on the proper ratio of zinc to copper in all these sites.[4]

"What does this mean?" asks Dr. Bland. "There are two direct relationships between zinc and copper nutrition and thyroid status. One is to the production of T4 and, potentially, to T3 and to the metabolism of these hormones in the cells where their activity will be used."

Dr. Bland reminds medical doctors that there are at least two ways to approach the patient with the symptoms of hypothyroidism.

"One way is the pharmacological approach, supplying larger doses of thyroid hormone through supplement. The second is normalizing the pituitary-thyroid and peripheral cell system by restoring the zinc-copper status in the individual deficient in these trace minerals."[5]

Such approaches often return the slipping male to full sexual potential, as many doctors who are experienced in thyroid hormone and trace mineral replacement are aware.

Hypothyroidism can diminish sexuality directly and indirectly. Fatigue and low endurance reduce both men and women to the survival level, where sexual activity plunges to the bottom of the priority list. Sex life automatically improves when general health is better.

Sex drive, potency and sexual sensitivity and enjoyment rise with a normal thyroid or one which is adequately supplemented. In hypothyroidism, insufficient pituitary hormone is synthesized and, as a result, the level of the sex hormone testosterone is low. Brain levels of dopamine are also low, which further diminishes sexual desire. Animal experiments show that thyroid hormones administered to the hypothyroid raise dopamine to normal levels.

Sluggish blood flow to the sex organs in hypothyroidism also can lessen sexual performance, as it can in atherosclerosis (narrowing of the arteries), a condition encouraged by subnormal thyroid function. (Atherosclerosis and hypothyroidism will be covered extensively in several later chapters.)

Hypoglycemia, whose symptoms are similar to those of hypothyroidism, often is present in the latter condition, resulting in zero energy and not much interest in sex.

One cause of hypertension, or high blood pressure, is hypothyroidism. Males who take hypertensive drugs over a protracted period sometimes lose their sex drive. Addiction to alcohol, narcotics and tobacco can also neutralize sex drive.

As in the case of Clayton, stress of various types can result in lower sex drive. An experiment with young male soldiers under the severe physical strain of a five-day combat course without sleep was reported in the *European Journal of Applied Physiology*.[6] After the first twenty-four hours, one of the thyroid hormones, thyroxine (T4), increased (apparently to compensate for stress). However, the other thyroid hormone, triiodothyronine (T3), did not. Within forty-eight hours, T4 had declined to normal, and T3 had gone lower.

The blood serum level of TSH went down throughout the experiment. Other hormones related to sexuality, prolactin and testosterone, also declined. Sleep helped reverse downtrends, particularly in prolactin and testosterone. Thyroid hormone production did not respond as readily. This experiment, in almost complete agreement with a previous study, points out the harmful effects of physical stress on general health and sexuality.

A less obvious stressor in many instances is low thyroid function. Sidney C. Werner, M.D., coeditor of *The Thyroid*, one of the most respected books in its field, states that sexual urge and potency are definitely reduced in extreme hypothyroidism.[7]

Among authorities who claim that decreased sexual drive is the most common reproductive abnormality of hypothyroid men is Peter Singer, M.D., Associate Clinical Professor of Medicine and Director, Thyroid Disease Diagnosis Center, Hospital of the Good Samaritan, Los Angeles.[8]

This, too, has been my repeated experience with patients. In psychological circles, it has been the custom to say that impotence is "all in the mind." Don't you believe it. It is also in the glands, starting with the thyroid. That is also where over-concern and immobilizing fears about potency may originate, as well as a host of emotional problems in areas other than sex.

MIND AND EMOTIONS: THE THYROID CONNECTION

*E*xhaustion and lack of endurance are not the only handi-caps of many untreated hypothyroids grimly trying to compete in the real world. To these must be added emotional problems, of which these individuals are sometimes not even aware.

The late Roy G. Hoskins, M.D., an eminent endocrinologist, found that even in seemingly mild cases of myxedema, there is an underlying irritability and hostility, in addition to mental and physical sluggishness.[1] In another common type of hypothyroidism, Dr. Hoskins noted a chip-on-the-shoulder attitude, an abnormal responsiveness to petty annoyances, but not necessarily the usual overweight or sluggishness. A state of general fatigue exists, along with "general poor health and, particularly, lack of endurance often designated chronic nervous exhaustion—and inability to endure physical or mental strain."

Dr. Hoskins referred to findings of endocrinologist H. F. Stoll, who discovered the following characteristics in "chronic hypothyroid invalidism": irritability, lying, suspiciousness, delusions, retarded ability to think, inability to concentrate, introversion and failing memory. Even mild to moderate stress can tilt the delicate balance of the low thyroid person and cause acute anxiety or depression. Such events as marriage, birth of a first child, a financial reverse, new job responsibilities can bring on greater energy depletion, headaches, temper tantrums, diarrhea or constipation, according to Dr. Stoll.

A study of twenty untreated hypothyroids by Dr. Martha Schon of the Neuropsychiatric Service at Memorial Hospital in New York City revealed such emotional traits as fatigue, nervousness, irritability, contrariness and temper explosions, which made it easy to mistake them for neurotics. She noted a major difference, however. Genuine neurotics blame others or circumstances for their problems. Low thyroid persons will generally accept responsibility for their emotional conduct.[2]

Dr. Schon found that with thyroid supplementation, almost all physical and emotional symptoms lessened or disappeared. Patients developed a sense of wellbeing and integration of personality. Apparently sub-clinical hypothyroidism can remain latent for years and not show itself in emotional or mental symptoms until after severe stress. A number of my patients have had this experience. Dr. Schon made the same discovery, observing that mental pressures with which patients could not cope brought on hypothyroidism.

Postpartum depression (the blues experienced by some women after delivery of a baby) may be attributable to low thyroid condition. That hypothyroidism can cause mild to severe neuroses and psychoses is not a new discovery.

Let us remember that Sigmund Freud, the father of psychoanalysis, predicted that some day a biologic or physiologic therapy would prove more effective in coping with emotional illness than psychotherapy. Carl Jung agreed.[3]

In the 1920s, Dr. Karl Mayer, a German scientist, demonstrated the power of thyroid extract to act as a biochemical psychiatrist on a patient no livelier than a block of ice—and equally silent—and normalize him.

More recently, successful use of thyroid hormone and vitamin therapy on psychiatric "rejects"—patients virtually unimproved with psychoanalysis—convinced Dr. Nathan Masor that conventional psychiatry needed biochemical backing.

Edward R. Pinckney, M.D., and Cathey Pinckney, authors of *The Fallacy of Freud and Psychoanalysis*, agree that unless the physical requirements for thyroid hormone are satisfied, psychiatric techniques will not help.

According to the Pinckneys,

> All too often, thyroid disease will manifest itself through nothing but behavioral symptoms. Neurotic actions may be the sole result of too little or too much thyroid, and the taking of a few inexpensive pills each day can produce instant normality in someone who seems to have a mental illness. Compare this type of treatment with years and years of costly lying on a couch, trying to uncover some infantile sexual frustration.
>
> But thyroid disease is not the only illness that indicates neurotic behavior. Patients with lung cancer repeatedly show marked hostility reaction. Infectious diseases, pelvic inflammations and even enlarged arteries have produced the very symptoms the psychoanalysts claim are due to unresolved sexual problems that began in childhood. What is contradictory to the Freudian doctrine is the fact that once an organic diagnosis is made and treated, there is an immediate disappearance of all neurotic behavior.[4]

An investigator at the University of North Carolina, Dr. P. C. Whybrow, studied a group of patients with severe mental disturbances who seemed excellent candidates for typical psychiatric treatment.[5] One of them was a woman whose son had been killed in a head-on car collision many years before and who constantly said that it would have been better if she had been the one killed. She had recurring dreams of reclaiming him from his grave by digging him up with her bare hands. All day long she heard her son calling to her. Considering herself a heavy burden for her family, she often entertained thoughts of suicide.

Another woman, plagued with insomnia, experienced vivid,

horrifying dreams when she did sleep—the death of her son and the mutilation of other family members. "I'm losing my mind," she insisted to family and doctors.

Both serious cases were quickly cleared up and the patients returned to normal behavior after thyroid treatment, thanks to enlightened psychiatrists.

Dr. Whybrow also found that hypothyroidism often manifests itself in two mental symptoms that are severe handicaps in daily living: poor recent memory and difficulty in concentrating. A Georgetown University study discovered these very symptoms in more than half of 109 cases of hypothyroidism.[6]

The most extreme form of hypothyroidism, myxedema, which is four to five times more common in women than in men, exaggerates mental shortcomings. Thinking, remembering and reacting occur in slow motion, if at all. A need to concentrate often puts the person to sleep. As one recovered patient told me, "In myxedema, thinking results in non-thinking. Mental effort is next to impossible. One is just a super-vegetable."

Dr. Masor reports that in even less extreme hypothyroidism, thinking is slow and memory impaired, often compounding emotional conditions such as listlessness, restlessness, irritability, a paranoid tendency, easy fatigue and miscellaneous body pains.[7] The fact that these symptoms melt away with appropriate daily thyroid therapy indicates that, in most cases, they are probably due to hypothyroidism.

In addition to supplementation with thyroid hormone, the diet should supply all essential nutrients. Lack of any B vitamins—particularly thiamine (B1) and cyanocobalamin (B12)—can slow thinking, cause memory lapses and irritability, as studies of semi-starved prisoners-of-war have revealed. On the other hand, supplying subjects in starvation experiments with missing B-complex vitamins, with accent on B1 and B12, brought about enhanced thinking and remembering, among other positive results.

In a double-blind experiment with matched-ability children, Dr. Ruth Flinn Herrell added just 2 mg of vitamin B1 to the daily diet of one group and a placebo to that of the second group. At the end of the study, the first group's mental and physical abilities rose from 7 to 87 percent. Those of the other group remained almost the same.[8]

An article in the *British Medical Journal* by Dr. J. MacDonald

Holmes, which cited various experiments, revealed that a deficiency of vitamin B12 brought on devastating mental and emotional symptoms such as difficulty in thinking and remembering, confusion, mood disorders, agitated depression, paranoia, delusions, visual and auditory hallucinations, maniacal behavior and epilepsy.[9]

Along with good nutrition, aerobic exercise encourages brain and memory function, says Professor Robert Rivera, a memory expert and speech teacher at Valley College in Van Nuys, California. Professor Rivera has found that more efficient blood and oxygen circulation to the brain can cause a significant increase in a person's I.Q.—as much as thirty points.

You may be able to validate Professor Rivera's findings by trying these simple exercises. First, you inhale for eight counts, hold your breath for twelve counts, then exhale for ten counts. He recommends repeating this exercise ten times. (Warning! If you feel dizzy, stop exercising at once!)

Second, you practice sitting up erectly at work and improve posture by standing and flattening yourself against a wall, then stretching. If the experiment is successful, you should observe a new sense of vigor, wellbeing and clarity of thinking.

The importance of oxygen to brain function is underscored by the fact that the grey matter, where thinking is done, uses one-quarter of our oxygen intake. Arterial blood of the brain must have an oxygen saturation of 90 percent for efficient thinking, according to Dr. Masor. If it is reduced to 85 percent, the ability for fine concentration and fine muscular coordination decreases. Reduce it to 74 percent, and faulty judgment results.[10] Such oxygen deprivation may also lead to emotional instability. Further oxygen reduction causes the nervous system to be depressed. Complete oxygen starvation for more than four minutes will often contribute to irreversible brain damage.

Hypothyroidism can cause oxygen deprivation in the brain in numerous ways: by impeding blood circulation (slowing the delivery of oxygen and nutrients); by slowing the rate of oxidation (burning) of food (glucose) to nourish brain cells; by depressing production of blood cells; by contributing to atherosclerosis (narrowing of arteries); and by limiting the amount of blood that reaches the brain. Dr. Masor points out that narrowing of vital brain arterioles by even one-sixteenth of their calibre can limit oxygen supply and bring about mental and emotional disturbances.

How hypothyroidism depresses blood cell production (and can actually contribute to a form of anemia) has been covered in detail in Chapter 4. How subnormal thyroid function encourages atherosclerosis will be explained in later chapters on heart and artery diseases.

Over and above contributing to disturbances of thought and memory processes, hypothyroidism may cause severe emotional changes, which, unfortunately, may be misdiagnosed as psychiatric disorders and treated unnecessarily with powerful drugs (some of them habit-forming) and hospitalization. One of its most serious, persistent and widespread consequences is depression, the subject of the next chapter.

8

A NEW LOOK AT DEPRESSION

*D*epressed persons are more likely to get relief from thyroid supplementation than from warmed-over psychotherapy.

New evidence that thyroid insufficiency is at the root of much depression and fatigue was announced by Mark Gold, M.D., and his associates at a conference on affective illness at Friends Hospital in Philadelphia.[1] In examining 350 inpatients and 44 outpatients at Fair Oaks Hospital, Summit, New Jersey, Dr. Gold found a "significant incidence of low-level hypothyroidism," convincing him that depression is often the first sign of low-level thyroid failure which is not detected by the usual thyroid function tests. Traditional blood tests for thyroid function in depressed patients revealed only 10 percent hypothyroids. Ninety percent of the depressed who were clinically hypothyroid showed normal thyroid blood tests.

Dr. Gold discovered that, when untreated, hypothyroidism became increasingly severe in a very short time. Early diagnosis and treatment led to a desirable reduction in depression. It is imperative to evaluate all psychiatric patients for hypothyroidism, Dr. Gold feels, because new data show that if thyroid function is reduced by 10 percent, brain thyroid function is diminished by a corresponding amount. A slowdown of the thyroid, even if we remain normal, will cause some changes in the brain. It doesn't surprise Dr. Gold that hypothyroids appear to be psychiatric patients.

He also explained that more than 10 percent of patients who visit psychiatrists with depression have a condition called asymptomatic autoimmune thyroiditis, an ailment in which the immune system attacks thyroid gland tissue, causing inflammation and under-function of the organ. As researchers are now finding, asymptomatic autoimmune thyroiditis does in fact have symptoms, one of which is depression. However, most cases of depression are caused by simple hypothyroidism. A letter to me from a patient who had suffered from depression of unsuspected origin for decades expresses the anguish that many such persons have in common.

My depression started when I was seventeen. The doctor ordered a basal metabolism test, which turned out to be − 10, a little low. He prescribed one grain of thyroid. I took it for a year and felt better.

Then I went into nurses' training and discontinued thyroid; I don't remember why. When I was thirty, the depression came back, along with low energy, but I never sought help. I didn't realize what was wrong.

I'm married and have two children but never seem to have enough energy to do anything except take care of the children. In my late forties, I lost interest in everything, just dragging around, feeling low and blue. I was little more than a vegetable. I couldn't have cared less if I woke up the next day.

Finally, a doctor diagnosed me as having depression. I had a series of shock treatments and several mood-elevating drugs. Then, when my doctor died, I couldn't find another doctor to help me. I struggled along with periods of mild depression and very low energy.

About three years ago, I heard Dr. Broda Barnes on a radio talk show, discussing hypothyroidism and his test. Later, I asked my new doctor for a thyroid function test, which proved negative. He refused to prescribe thyroid.

All my life, I had noticed that I ran a subnormal temperature but hadn't thought much about it. One day I took my early morning temperature and found it low. My sister who was visiting had some thyroid pills, and I started taking a small dose. Almost immediately my depression lifted and my energy rose, too.

Then I heard Dr. Barnes on the air again, this time as your guest, and I decided to see you. I'm so glad I did. As you know, my basal temperature was low and you gave me thyroid. Many, many thanks for seeing through my problems, for realizing I was not a mental patient who needed more shock treatments, mood-elevating drugs or psychoanalysis. I feel great now!

Within a month, her fifteen-year-long depression was eliminated. It saddened me that this well-meaning person could not get simple, safe, low-cost thyroid to help her and instead was subjected to two series of arduous, expensive and unnecessary shock treatments, which could do nothing to compensate for her shortage of thyroid hormones.

I wish I could say that this is a rare case. However, many of my patients are over age fifty and, as children, teenagers or even adults, had had thyroid supplementation which was cut off when they or their doctor moved. During the 1950s, blood tests came into vogue and were not always positive for hypothyroidism. Patients were told that they no longer needed thyroid, and most of them suffered decades of unnecessary depression, anxiety and physical discomfort and limitation.

In fairness to the doctors of the 1950s and 1960s, the Barnes Basal Temperature Test was not then widely known, although Dr. Barnes's landmark paper on this test had already been published in the *Journal of the American Medical Association*. Today, however, there is little excuse for being unaware of it and its validity.

Despite the Basal Temperature Test's accuracy in revealing hypothyroidism, there is a minute percentage of cases which are too subtle to be detectable by this method. Not long ago, a patient in her early thirties, whom I'll call Phyllis, took the Barnes test and registered 97.8 degrees the first day and 97.7 the second day. She tried again on the third day and showed a temperature of 97.7. This averaged out to less than a tenth of a point below normal. Yet this woman had a serious problem with depression. She admitted that frequently, in the electronic assembly department which she supervises, she almost burst into tears at the slightest frustration, something she couldn't afford to do without reducing her stature and jeopardizing her position, which she had worked hard for fifteen years to attain.

I asked all the right questions. Had she gone through severe stresses—the death of a spouse, relative or close friend, a revolutionary change on the job, the break-up of a love affair?

"No, doctor. Nothing like that," she responded.

"Anything seem radically wrong physically?" I asked.

"No. I'm a little more tired than usual. That's all."

"Are you always depressed, or is it intermittent?"

"I do have good days and weeks, sometimes months. But it's worse this winter than last."

I darted a glance at the calendar (sometimes you need a calendar to determine the season, because winters in northern California are quite mild) and realized that Phyllis had given me the clue I needed. She was definitely hypothyroid, despite her body temperature reading. Her deepest depression was in the winter season, when temperatures were ten to fifteen degrees cooler than in fall or summer. Colder weather makes it necessary for the thyroid to step up the burning of fuel. This slight change accented her hypothyroidism, mild as it was.

I explained the problem to Phyllis, who agreed to take a grain of thyroid daily. She never regretted it. Within three weeks, her depression began to recede, and two months later she said, "It's hard for me to remember not feeling okay. My energy level is great. It's wonderful to be a human being again."

Like Phyllis's case, Benton's had certain mystifying aspects at first. A certified public accountant who owned his own firm, Benton plunged into deep depression near the middle of April—the end of income tax season. That was understandable, because of the extreme stress he was under at tax deadline time. However, it was now the end of May, and the depression had grown worse. Certainly a person in good health would have recovered already.

Benton's basal temperature was just a shade under the normal 97.8. A complete medical history and physical examination done at that time were inconclusive. Because of his symptoms, however, I decided to start him on a half grain of desiccated thyroid. Even this small amount of natural thyroid medication worked wonders.

Thyroid hormone has been studied intensively in depressed patients. In one double-blind controlled study, just 25 mcg of thyroid daily enhanced the anti-depressant action of the drug imipramine by 50 percent. Forty mcg was even more effective with imipramine.[2]

Of course, not all depression is caused by hypothyroidism. Poor nutrition is another major unsuspected cause. In such cases, dietary counseling and nutritional supplements banish depression almost miraculously. Many nutrition-oriented doctors have successfully used the amino acid tryptophan to combat depression. A breakthrough double-blind controlled study on this subject was reported in *Lancet*.[3] Patients taking 6 grams a day of tryptophan showed significant improvement with no side effects. Others taking imipramine improved faster but suffered undesirable side effects.

The amount of tryptophan ingested in this study would have been impossible to obtain from diet alone, since one would have had to eat more than a pound of soybeans to obtain 6 grams of this amino acid.

An unsuspected cause of depression in women is the taking of oral contraceptive pills. When a patient is depressed and on the Pill, I have her change to another form of contraception as soon as possible and treat her immediately for B-complex deficiency, particularly vitamin B6, known to be depleted in chronic users of oral contraceptives. If there is, in fact, a B-complex deficiency, a B-complex vitamin including at least 50 mg of vitamin B6 usually helps to dispel depression.

Sometimes when the lack of B complex is caused by the use of birth control pills, severe depression follows childbirth (postpartum depression). This condition usually responds to B-complex vitamins.

The trace mineral lithium is often thought to be an excellent treatment for depression. Actually, it may worsen depression, because it interferes with thyroid function. On the basis of a thorough study, P. L. Rabin and D. C. Evans of Vanderbilt University School of Medicine verify this fact in the *Journal of Clinical Psychiatry:* "... goiter formation and hypothyroidism are not infrequent following lithium therapy...."[4]

Unfortunately, hypothyroidism is still not widely enough recognized as a major cause of depression. It would be a mistake, however, to consider subnormal thyroid function and nutritional deficiences as the *only* causes.

9

MEDICAL LOOK-ALIKES:
HYPOGLYCEMIA AND
HYPOTHYROIDISM

*A*nother heavyweight contributor to depression is hypoglycemia (low blood sugar), an insidious disorder with many
emotional and physical symptoms, the best known of which
is deep fatigue.[1]

In a survey of 600 hypoglycemia patients, Dr. Stephen Gyland
found that depression ranked fifth among their complaints and
was experienced by 77 percent of his subjects.

It is understandable why hypoglycemia causes a long list of
emotional ailments in addition to depression: forgetfulness,
insomnia, anxiety, confusion, antisocial behavior, crying jags,
lack of concentration and assorted phobias. When our blood
sugar is too low, our brains are deprived of glucose, the only

fuel they can use. This starvation brings on the symptoms which are misdiagnosed as neuroses.

Hypoglycemia results mainly from how the body handles—or mishandles—sugar, rather than from the amount of sugar in the blood at a given time. When a normal person takes in a simple refined carbohydrate, such as table sugar, the blood level of sugar rises. Then the hormone insulin, secreted by the pancreas, soon brings down blood sugar to the fasting level.

When the hypoglycemic ingests sugar, however, the pancreas suffers shock and over-reacts, discharging so much insulin into the blood that sugar is removed too rapidly, creating a glucose deficit. Secondary results from prolonged hyperinsulinism are an off-balance nervous system, over-stimulated adrenal glands often stressed in the process of elevating blood sugar level, and an eventual shortage of blood sugar-elevating hormones—adrenal, glucagon and a pituitary gland hormone.

From the standpoint of symptoms, hypoglycemia is like hypothyroidism. Dr. Broda Barnes feels that these disorders are almost as closely related as Siamese twins, and his reasons make good sense.

He told me how he happened to stumble onto this connection. A legal secretary, prior to being treated by Dr. Barnes, passed out in her office, apparently from a heart attack, and was rushed to a hospital's intensive care unit. Three days of comprehensive, sophisticated tests revealed nothing organically wrong. She had other blackouts, more siren-screaming races to intensive care, more tests, more medical costs and still no diagnosis firm enough to support a therapy program. Then she found a physician who understood the biochemical basis for hypoglycemia and put her on a high-protein, low-carbohydrate diet, which brought about some improvement. However, she was not completely satisfied. She was referred to Dr. Barnes, who observed that she showed many symptoms of hypothyroidism, including a subnormal basal temperature.

With natural thyroid therapy, she recovered rapidly and never again experienced a blackout. As Dr. Barnes put it, "The light suddenly dawned. If she were hypothyroid and hypoglycemic, might not the two ailments occur together in many individuals?"

He explains his theory in the following terms: "A sluggish liver results from subnormal thyroid activity. During periods of stress, the liver can't produce enough sugar from protein. Then hypoglycemia occurs. Thyroid therapy stimulates the liver to normal function, and hypoglycemia usually disappears."

Dr. Barnes cites three bits of evidence of sluggish liver in hypothyroidism. For more than one hundred years, researchers have noted that myxedema patients (those with extremely low thyroid function) have a yellowish skin color, caused by too much carotene in the blood. A liver low in thyroid hormone has difficulty converting carotene to vitamin A, which is colorless. Thyroid therapy stimulates liver function, and the yellowish skin color vanishes.

Another piece of evidence is that blood cholesterol is usually high in hypothyroidism. Thyroid supplementation lowers cholesterol, because the liver is once again working normally, turning excess cholesterol into bile salts, which are discharged in the bile.

The third piece of evidence is that the sluggish liver of the hypothyroid stores glucose more slowly than a normal organ. Therefore, the blood level of sugar may register high during a fasting glucose tolerance test. The patient may also spill glucose in the urine and for these reasons will probably be labeled a "prediabetic."

"When such an individual is put on thyroid therapy, the liver begins to function properly and the glucose tolerance test is normal," says Dr. Barnes. "Many so-called prediabetics are really hypothyroids. This accounts for the fact that so few of them ever become diabetics."

Blood sugar levels are also closely associated with correct functioning of the adrenals, two ductless glands which perch on top of the kidneys and produce the hormone adrenalin. Most of us are familiar with one essential function of the adrenals: triggering the discharge of liver glucose (stored as glycogen) into the bloodstream to give us instant energy in the face of danger. These key glands also secrete and release other essential hormones. The major ones are cortisol (hydrocortisone) and cortisone, both glucocorticoids related to liver sugar.

A study included in perhaps the most prestigious textbook on the thyroid gland, *The Thyroid*, edited by Sidney C. Werner, M.D., and Sidney H. Ingbar, M.D., gives a clue as to how hypothyroidism influences at least one important function of the adrenal glands related to blood sugar.

One of cortisol's most significant functions is stimulating the liver's production of glycogen. An experiment cited in *The Thyroid* shows that hypothyroids secrete cortisol at a reduced rate. This means that liver sugar is produced more slowly. Treatment with thyroid hormone normalizes cortisol metabolism.

The Werner-Ingbar book states that hypothyroidism in animals sometimes causes adrenal atrophy (wasting away), which could undermine every function of this gland. The findings in human beings have not been so conclusive. What is well established, however, is that the thyroid gland is closely associated with blood sugar levels, although all the reasons for this are not as yet known.

Dr. Barnes adds a footnote in regard to hypothyroidism and hypoglycemia. In more than four decades as a medical doctor, he has treated more than 5,000 patients for the symptoms of subnormal thyroid function and has not seen one case of hypoglycemia develop. He does admit, however, that only in the last two decades has this disorder become well enough known for him and other medical doctors to be alert to it.

Patients who have come to Dr. Barnes with hypoglycemia have usually responded to thyroid therapy with no change in diet. My experience in this regard varies slightly. In many instances, my patients have overcome low blood sugar with thyroid hormones. However, I have also had excellent response from diet.

My dietary approach to this disorder is purposely uncomplicated. First, I explain to patients that a simple carbohydrate wastes no time going through the digestive process and into the bloodstream—foods such as sugar, corn syrup and glucose, for example. Complex refined carbohydrates like bread, cornstarch, flour, white rice and potato starch are not quite so fast. Complex unrefined carbohydrates—legumes, nuts, seeds, vegetables, whole grains, wholegrain cereals—are slower, followed by proteins and then fats, the slowest.

A mixed diet—some complex carbohydrates, protein, and a little fat—assures gradual release of sugar into the bloodstream. The pancreas is protected from sugar-shock. Ample protein from meat, fish, poultry, eggs or dairy products and low-carbohydrate vegetables and fruit make an ideal diet for the hypoglycemic. Most fruits and vegetables can be included, although, I usually eliminate those in the 20 percent carbohydrate bracket: bananas, sweet cherries, fresh figs, grape juice and prunes, as well as kidney, lima and navy beans, corn and hominy. Fruits and vegetables to be eaten sparingly are the following in the 15 percent carbohydrate group: apples, apricots, blueberries, sour cherries, grapes, loganberries, pears, pineapple, plums and raspberries, as well as artichokes, parsnips and peas.

Some authorities on hypoglycemia recommend from five to seven small meals daily, rather than the traditional three. By mixing food groups, I find that most patients can manage hypoglycemia well with three meals, but I suggest that they experiment. If more small meals work for them, I urge them to follow such a routine.

So much for low blood sugar. Next we will deal with high blood sugar.

10

DIABETES—A PREVENTABLE DISEASE

A little knowledge about diabetes, a blood sugar disorder that plagues almost 11 million Americans, will go a long way to prevent it and—for those already diabetic—to lessen this ailment's health-destroying effects, reduce dependency on insulin and dramatically decrease the chances of sometimes fatal diabetic complications.

Telltale symptoms of diabetes are excessive thirst, frequent and copious urination, constant hunger, extreme systemic acidity, rapid weight loss, severe itching, fatigue, weakness and, above all, high sugar level in the blood and urine.

Elevated blood sugar is due to a breakdown of the body's energy use system. Glucose, a simple sugar derived from food, is our major fuel for heat and energy. Although blood circulation carries glucose to all of our body cells, it cannot penetrate the cell walls unless it is attached to molecules of the pancreatic hormone insulin. In an insulin shortage, much blood sugar accumulates and circulates helplessly, finally passing into the kidneys for excretion in the urine.

On its way into our stomach, the food we eat triggers the release of insulin into the bloodstream. Most blood sugar is used for energy. However, some enters the liver to be changed into glycogen and is stored there and in the muscles for use according to our body's needs. If we over-eat, the excess calories are converted by our body into fat deposits.

Insulin is secreted by the pancreas, a yellowish glandular organ lying horizontally under the stomach. This hormone is formed in a part of the pancreas called the islets of Langerhans, which contain the all-important alpha and beta cells. Alpha cells secrete a hormone called glucagon, which, when called upon, raises the blood sugar level by activating the conversion of stored glycogen into glucose. The beta cells secrete the hormone insulin, which lowers blood sugar level. The outputs of the alpha and beta cells are supposed to be in balance. In the diabetic, however, insulin is often in short supply, for reasons which will be discussed later.

In addition to these secretions, the pancreas excretes proteolytic enzymes, molecules which help create the proper pH (acid-base) environment in the digestive system for these proteolytic enzymes to function. They break down proteins into body-usable amino acids.

Many theories explain how diabetes develops. Perhaps the most accepted one is that repeated and heavy intake of sugar causes the body's energy system to become defective. Sugar entering the bloodstream signals the beta cells to secrete more insulin, keeping them in production until the glucose level drops to normal. Repeated assaults by large amounts of sugar force the pancreas to work overtime in producing insulin. Eventually, it becomes exhausted and production slumps.

In some instances, however, insulin shortage may not be the problem. Experiments by Dr. Walter Mertz, chief of the U.S. Department of Agriculture's Vitamin and Mineral Research Division, indicate that a shortage of chromium can bring on diabetes.[1]

To escort glucose through cell walls, insulin needs the close cooperation of infinitesimal amounts of chromium as a catalyst. Most maturity-onset diabetes (i.e., in mid-years to advanced age) results from a diet of chromium-poor processed foods and could probably be prevented by use of chromium-rich foods such as brewer's yeast, beef liver, chicken, various meats, and whole grains.

Some scientists state that diabetes is caused by the islets of Langerhans' release of pro-insulin, rather than biologically usuable insulin. For unexplained reasons, this "not quite" form of the hormone never goes through its final chemical changes.

Research at the University of Texas Southwestern Medical School suggests that diabetes is a two-hormone disorder brought about by a shortage of insulin and an excess of blood-sugar-raising glucagon.

Authorities agree that genes predispose us toward diabetes, that children born of at least one diabetic parent are more likely to be diabetic than those from nondiabetic parents. They may be diabetes-prone because their pancreas does not function properly or because their cell receptors do not take up glucose efficiently.

While admitting the importance of the inheritance factor, other authorities indicate that innumerable environmental factors, including food selection, preparation, consumption and repetition, as well as stresses, are probably even more important. One group within this school of thought holds that heredity is given more weight than it deserves, because researchers gather their statistics without considering that poor diet and other negative environmental conditions passed down from generation to generation are also a key part of physical ailments which appear to be strictly hereditary.

It is now well known that one of the adrenal gland hormones, epinephrine, released into the bloodstream in fight-or-flight situations, increases free fatty acids in the blood and turns off the release of insulin. Unresolved and continued stress can therefore upset the balance of pancreas hormones and bring on diabetes.

Another kind of stress, obesity, invites diabetes. At a conference on diabetes mellitus and obesity, Dr. W. John H. Butterfield, Professor of Medicine at Guys Hospital in London, revealed an amazing similarity in how the body handles carbohydrates in diabetes and in gross overweight.[2]

Dr. Butterfield described his experiment on comparative cell glucose uptake of three groups of test subjects: juvenile diabetics, maturity-onset diabetics and normal controls.

Juvenile diabetics absorbed no sugar in their cells, a strong indication that they were short on internally secreted insulin. Glucose uptake of older diabetic patients and obese normal subjects was similar. Lean controls took up more sugar than plump ones.

Obese subjects handled carbohydrates almost like diabetics, said Dr. Butterfield. As obesity progresses, less and less insulin reaches the insulin-responsive muscles, so less and less glucose uptake occurs there, making it necessary for more and more insulin to be formed. When obesity increases to certain proportions, the pancreas can't keep up production of insulin to meet demand, and hyperglycemia results. Reversible-obesity diabetes, then, adds up to a breakdown of the body's insulin-glucose economy.

Another significant insight of Dr. Butterfield's about the diabetes-proneness of obese people is that body fat competes with muscle for insulin, and fat wins. Then carbohydrates are changed into more fat.

Both obese and lean diabetics usually reduce blood fats and the need for insulin on a high fiber diet. This is the conclusion reached by James Anderson, M.D., of the University of Kentucky, a long-time researcher in high-fiber diets—those containing large amounts of raw foods, fruits, vegetables, whole grain breads, bran, nuts and seeds. The most marked improvement was in obese patients who lost the greatest amount of weight. Excellent high-fiber foods are spinach, prunes, corn, fresh peas, blackberries, sweet potatoes, apples, wholewheat bread, potatoes, broccoli, almonds, raisins, zucchini, plums and kidney beans.

Associate Professor Somasundaram Addanki of the Ohio State University College of Medicine agrees with the need for a high-fiber diet in managing *and* preventing diabetes. However, he goes farther.[3] Ninety percent of diabetes-prone individuals can avoid this disorder by not eating "the typical high-fat, high-sugar and low-fiber diet consumed in western countries," he writes in the journal *Preventive Medicine*.[4]

Professor Addanki speaks from personal experience as well as in-depth research on this subject. A diabetic who married a diabetic, he says that he and his wife did not develop diabetes until they left their native India and started eating American foods. He does not agree that heredity is a primary factor. Only 8 percent of cases can be attributed to heredity, as comparative studies in Africa and Japan indicate. These findings relieved Addanki about the future of his children.

Further data that the typical American diet exerts the most powerful influence on development of diabetes emerge from a comparison of Japanese living in Japan and others who moved to Hawaii. After eating western food in Hawaii, they invariably developed diabetes in greater numbers.

A biochemist and nutritionist, Addanki explains why the poor American diet turns healthy individuals into diabetics. Fatty, sugary, low-fiber foods stimulate certain intestinal bacteria to produce excessive estrogen, a female hormone. It is also probable that an enzyme in fatty tissues unites with testosterone, the male hormone, to synthesize more estrogen. Estrogen desensitizes skeletal muscles to insulin action. As more weight is added, more estrogen is produced, more insulin is required to be effective, and there is greater stress on the pancreas, the insulin-producer, which wears out too soon.

The excess estrogen theory explains why obese adult men are often impotent, while women frequently experience a more powerful sexual drive. In a United Press International story explaining his theory, Professor Addanki admitted to six years of "diabetic impotence" before a change of diet brought him control over his disease. He advises all fat people to give up sugar, white flour and fatty foods if they want to avoid the risk of developing diabetes.

Another authority who has evidence that exhaustion of the pancreas underlies the development of diabetes is William H. Philpott, M.D. A prominent clinical ecologist, he has a different explanation as to how this happens, and he elaborates it in an illuminating book, *Victory Over Diabetes*, written with Dwight K. Kalita, Ph.D.[5] He observes that the pancreas secretes a substance called somastatin, which acts as a balancing mechanism between the organ's other hormones, glucagon (blood-sugar-raising) and insulin (blood-sugar-lowering).

"Obviously, a proper harmony must exist between these various functions of the pancreas to avoid diabetes," he writes. "If we were to stop at this point with our examination of the pancreas, we might conclude, as has been done by many physicians, that diabetes is a simple matter of controlling high blood sugar levels by the daily injection of insulin.

"However, as we have already seen, although high blood sugar levels may indeed be controlled by the use of insulin, the associated killing complications of diabetes are not easily dealt with. There is, in fact, medical evidence ... that daily injections of insulin may, in part, actually be responsible for some of the many severe cardiovascular and cerebrovascular complications associated with this disease." (Complications of this disorder will be dealt with in detail in a later chapter.)

Dr. Philpott explains that pancreas-made insulin travels through the bloodstream to the liver, where at least half of it is used. The rest of the body needs only a small amount.

Insulin injected under the skin of the arm, leg or buttocks travels the entire peripheral circulatory system before reaching the liver, and much more insulin than is needed in the vascular system remains there. Compounding this problem is the fact that unless sufficient insulin is injected to satisfy the liver's requirements, a serious condition, ketoacidosis, will develop. Dr. Philpott feels that, under these conditions, hyperinsulinism is almost unavoidable and contributes to severe complications of diabetes.

Why should a natural substance such as insulin create problems? Dr. Philpott answers in the following terms: "... Dr. R. W. Stout, of Hammersmith Hospital in London, actually showed that when laboratory rats were given insulin intravenously, the insulin stimulated the synthesis of cholesterol in blood vessel walls.

"Other investigators have shown that when too much insulin is present in the blood, all kinds of *metabolic debris* can be found, including certain chemicals that are deposited on the insides of blood vessels that have been partly occluded [closed], as in arteriosclerosis."

No part of the body, including the pancreas, is necessarily exempt from this condition. Over and above injected insulin, other outside factors can undermine the pancreas, including chemicals in the environment and foods to which we may be allergic or hypersensitive.

The first organ to be influenced by exposure to ingested foods and chemicals, the pancreas, has the key task of turning these substances into forms usable by the body and also of protecting the body from negative reaction to them. Food allergens and harmful chemicals cause the pancreas to be overstimulated and overworked, and thus weaken it.

"All addictions, of course, whether they are foods of any kind, chemicals, tobacco and/or alcohol, eventually lead to pancreatic insufficiency of varying degrees," Dr. Philpott explains, "but what is important to realize is that most affected in pancreatic insufficiency of these types are the bicarbonate and enzyme productions of the organ...."

Let's look at what happens in pancreatic insufficiency. Added to a lessening ability to secrete insulin and glucagon, the pancreas produces inadequate amounts of pancreatic enzymes and bicarbonate, which threatens the proper functioning of the entire organ.

Unless the pancreas can make sufficient proteolytic enzymes to secrete into the intestines, proteins cannot be properly broken down into amino acids for body use. This leads to a deficiency of amino acids and a disastrous chain reaction. Proteolytic enzymes are made from amino acids. In a deficiency of amino acids, these enzymes will soon be deficient.

"With an amino acid deficiency, there is more than just a reduced enzyme production from the pancreas.... Insulin is composed of fifty-one amino acids. When these all-important building blocks of hormones are in short supply, the quality and quantity of insulin production actually begin to diminish. This, of course, can lead to a deficiency of insulin with the resulting effect of high blood sugar or diabetes," writes Dr. Philpott.

Subnormal function of the pancreas also causes diminished production of lipase, an enzyme essential to proper metabolism of fats. This causes a rise in free fatty acids in the bloodstream, which is encouragement for arteriosclerosis.

Still another complication from a deficient pancreas and its reduced production of proteolytic enzymes is that proteins are not properly digested into amino acids and large particles in the bloodstream lodge in the tissues. The body's immune system is immediately activated and it attacks these particles as undesirable aliens, causing inflammation and injury in the arteries or wherever else they lodge.

Dr. Philpott warns that cooking foods above 118 degrees Fahrenheit destroys digestive enzymes, putting an added burden on the pancreas, salivary glands, stomach and intestines to come "to the rescue and furnish digestive enzymes (protease for the proteins, lipase for fats and amylase for carbohydrates) to break down these substances.

"To do this repeatedly, the body must rob ... enzymes from other glands, muscles, nerves and the blood to help in its demanding digestive process. Eventually, the glands—and this includes the pancreas—develop deficiencies of enzymes, because they have been forced to work harder, due to the low level of enzymes in cooked food."

An experiment in the University of Minnesota's Department of Anatomy showed that rats fed an 80 percent cooked food diet for 155 days had an increase of pancreatic weight by 20 to 30 percent "with a corresponding decrease in digestive enzyme secretions. And what is true of animals is also true of man," writes Dr. Philpott.

Although the pancreas can manufacture enzymes, we must not overdraw on our enzyme potential.

"... The more we use our enzyme potential, the faster it is going to run out," he maintains. "When you eat food that is raw, the enzymes contained in the food immediately start breaking down the food ingested."

In other words, if you eat as much raw food as possible, you put less burden on your pancreas and extend its healthy life.

When pancreas function is diminished, production of bicarbonate is also reduced. This is a vital secretion, needed to increase the alkalinity of the small intestine.

"In pancreatic deficiencies, acute metabolic acidosis after the meal occurs," writes Dr. Philpott, "since the pancreatic bicarbonate, now undersupplied, has not neutralized acid from the stomach as it empties into the duodenum plus the small intestine.

"This reduction of proper bicarbonate levels in the pancreas results in a chain reaction whereby the pancreatic proteolytic enzymes, which are also secreted into the small intestine, and which need an alkaline medium in which to function best, are destroyed."

There is a wealth of additional helpful information in Dr. Philpott's *Victory Over Diabetes*, which is a book that every diabetic should have for ready reference.

Another stress on the pancreas not mentioned by Dr. Philpott is subnormal body temperature caused by hypothyroidism, particularly myxedema, and by less extreme subnormal thyroid function. This may be the reason why so many diabetics are also hypothyroid.

Some years ago, C. D. Eaton, M.D., of Detroit, published a revealing report, "Co-Existence of Hypothyroidism with Diabetes Mellitus," in *The Journal of the Michigan Medical Society.*[6] In studying hundreds of his diabetic patients, he found symptoms of hypothyroidism and diabetes to be similar—all but the carbohydrate metabolism disturbance in the latter. Symptoms in common were low energy, weakness, constipation, itching, sleepiness, high levels of blood fat, muscle pains, high susceptibility to infection, poor wound healing, early atherosclerosis, and gangrene. He discovered that hypothyroidism was far more frequent in diabetics than in non-diabetics.

Dr. Eaton observed that insulin controlled the blood sugar level in diabetics but did nothing to correct the other symptoms. Administration of small doses of natural thyroid did, however, as I will explain in a later chapter.

To summarize and accentuate the key points in this chapter, here are the principal ways to prevent diabetes or to lessen its effects and the chances of diabetic complications:

1. Refrain from eating refined sugar and other refined carbohydrates. (Remember that processed food products often contain hidden sugars. Read labels carefully.)

2. Make sure your diet includes some chromium-rich foods—brewer's yeast, beef liver, chicken, meat, and whole grains—because without chromium insulin cannot carry nutrients through the walls of your trillions of cells.

3. Try to avoid unnecessary stress, and make practical adjustments to that which is unavoidable. Stress slows down insulin production.

4. Exercise regularly.

5. Eat a high-fiber diet for reasons of general health but particularly to reduce chances of developing diabetes or of lessening the need for insulin.

6. Avoid becoming obese. Overweight individuals are prime targets for diabetes. (The next chapter deals with weight loss.)

7. Keep your pancreas healthy, not only by avoiding assaults of refined sugar which overwork this organ, but also by avoiding chemicals, tobacco and alcohol, and by eating more raw vegetables for their live enzymes. A steady diet of cooked foods can deplete the existing bank of digestive enzymes and harm the pancreas.

8. Be certain that your body temperature is normal and that you are not hypothyroid, a condition which places stress on the pancreas.

9. Remember that insulin can control blood sugar levels but does nothing to prevent complications of diabetes. Thyroid hormone can help in this regard.

11

OVERWEIGHT: HOW TO BE A GOOD LOSER!

Whoever first called the struggle to shed unwanted weight the Battle of the Bulge was guilty of a serious understatement. It seems more like the Hundred Years' War!

I am constantly besieged by patients whose best efforts at losing weight have been none too good. It is not surprising that they lose their fighting hearts. Many of them have been on every diet touted by best-selling books: high carbohydrate-low fat; high fiber; low carbohydrate-high protein; juices; fasts; and other regimes conceived by the profit-motivated human mind.

Some patients lose weight, but not for long. Sooner or later—usually sooner—they slip back into old eating habits, and the fat comes back bigger and better than ever. As one of those fortunate fellows who carry no more fat than a racing greyhound, I am going to give you a plan that keeps me slim and helps my patients reduce. My system doesn't promise as quick returns as best-seller regimes, but it does work. It starts with the underlying principles of encouraging good health and proper thyroid function, which are basic to efficient weight loss.

Most overweight individuals are undernourished and suffering from subclinical malnutrition. This condition doesn't always lead to immediate catastrophic illness, but it will lead to biochemical imbalance that may cause health problems and preclude weight loss. It is important to avoid incomplete and unbalanced diets. Temporary shedding of a few pounds is not worth the loss of good health.

We are all different and therefore require different quantities of the same essential nutrients to stay healthy. No matter how complete your diet appears, you can't get from it all the essential nutrients in proper amounts. You must therefore take nutritional supplements to maintain optimal health. You must be realistic about your food supply. On its trip from the ground to your gullet, your food may lose as much as 50 percent of some essential nutrients, even before it is processed.

In order to be in good health and to lose weight, you must have normal thyroid function—or appropriate supplementation—to realize full values from your food. Even if your diet contains all essential micronutrients in proper amounts, you may not be getting full nutritional benefit from it.

Food must be broken down and absorbed through the gastrointestinal mucosa. This process is inefficient in hypothyroidism. Next, food must be processed by pancreatic enzymes and converted by the liver in order to become biochemically active. (Assimilation is often faulty in hypothyroid patients.) Then food must be transported by the circulatory system to the sites of use at the cellular level and successfully enter the cell to provide nutritional fuel. Lack of certain nutrients retards the process.

After all this, wastes have to be efficiently eliminated from cells and carried by the circulatory system for detoxification by the kidneys and liver and thrown off by the bowels, urinary system, skin and lungs—all of which function below par in hypothyroid individuals.

In hypothyroidism, a decreased rate of oxygen use and a diminished rate of heat production translate into a decrease in metabolism and an inability to lose weight, no matter how hard we try. Administration of thyroid hormone restores both oxygen consumption and metabolic functioning to the hypothyroid individual.

Now comes a key fact. All dieters are familiar with the "sticking point"—the point at which the bathroom scale stubbornly refuses to go lower. In the hypothyroid, this is attributable to a worsening of the hypothyroidism, in which the body sets its thermostat lower.

Hypothyroidism does not make you fat. Dr. Barnes always points out that upwards of 40 percent of his hypothyroid patients are actually underweight. However, if you are overweight and hypothyroid, you will probably need to be taking thyroid hormone to facilitate the usefulness of any diet you are on.

Your doctor has probably told you that taking thyroid hormone to lose weight is an unnecessary placebo if you don't have low thyroid blood tests. Unfortunately, this is not the case. It is possible to be hypothyroid even with an adequate thyroid hormone output, because of biochemical differences in the receptor sites in our cells, and this condition will show up on the basal temperature test.

What can you do to lose weight? Follow the rules listed below.

1. Make sure your thyroid gland is functioning normally so that you can rule out hypothyroidism, a handicap to weight loss. Start with the Barnes Basal Temperature Test.

2. Eat frequent small meals from the four major food groups.

3. Increase your vegetable intake for all of its nutritional contributions, particularly live enzymes which help the digestion and absorption process, and added dietary bulk to speed up elimination.

4. Avoid refined carbohydrates, including sugar, white flour and white rice.

5. Avoid foods containing preservatives and artificial additives (coloring, flavoring, stabilizing and foaming).

6. Don't add salt to foods. Avoid restaurants which salt their menu items. Avoid sodium-containing additives such as MSG.

7. Avoid overcooked foods. Use leftover cooking liquids in soups and gravies.

8. Minimize your use of animal or saturated fats. Use only lean cuts of meat, trim off fat and remove fat-laden skin from chicken.

9. Don't use heated vegetable oils. Don't fry foods in oil. Heating vegetable oils and fats makes them as harmful to the body as animal fats and robs your system of essential fatty acids.

10. Get a hair analysis and a computerized nutritional evaluation. They will help to pinpoint deficiencies in your diet. Better yet, have a consultation with a physician who specializes in preventive health maintenance.

11. Improve your diet by taking nutritional supplements.

12. Add bulk to your diet to reduce your appetite. Glucomannan is a harmless fiber product which, if taken with at least eight ounces of water fifteen to twenty minutes before meals, will accomplish this and, in most instances, make you feel full without excess calories.

13. Check on evening primrose oil, an over-the-counter nutritional supplement sold at most nutrition centers which I have found helpful in weight reduction programs. Two capsules after each meal (or three times a day) is the recommended amount for adults.

14. Avoid diet beverages, dark teas (of the non-herbal variety), coffee and more than four to six ounces of fruit or vegetable juices at one sitting or more than one piece of raw fruit at a single meal.

15. Never starve yourself.

16. Get professional psychological counseling if you have had overweight problems for more than a year. Many individuals and families working to lose weight often unconsciously sabotage their own program for a variety of hidden reasons. A professional counselor can often unearth these problems. It is also difficult for some dieters to adjust to the success of their program, to becoming more attractive and more socially acceptable. Such conflicts can be brought to light by counseling and, after a few brief sessions, eliminated.

17. Remember, strictly vegetarian diets are notoriously deficient in micronutrients such as vitamin B12 and others; this has been mentioned in previous chapters. Such shortcomings must be corrected by dietary changes and nutritional supplementation.

18. Exercise aerobically (unless you are seriously ill or your doctor has advised against it). This is an essential part of any weight-control program. The best exercise that most of us can enjoy and participate in is brisk walking for fifteen to twenty minutes, three or four times a week.

19. Recognize that you are responsible for the success or failure of your weight control program. You notice that I did not include any rigid menus in this chapter for the simple reason that most of them don't work. We tend to revert to our old, established eating habits, no matter what diet we're on, because of ethnic likes and dislikes, mistrust of the new and inertia. More important than a set of menus is an awareness of nutritional principles on which you can build your own best diet based on your food likes and dislikes. If you eat small meals from all the essential food groups and eliminate junky, refined and convenience foods from your diet, you will almost always lose weight.

20. Don't expect perfection in following your diet. This can lead to depression if you slip. Remember, two steps forward and one step backward is better than the reverse. Strive to the best of your ability for moderation. Allow yourself to binge on rare occasions, if you consciously control when those occasions occur. If you can't do this, please reread number 16 and pay careful attention to number 21.

21. If you're following all of the previous suggestions and are still struggling to lose weight, you are probably suffering from food allergies, which often cause serious food addictions and weight gain. Food allergy and sensitivity were purposely not discussed in detail, because they fall outside the scope of this book. However, my own clinical experience indicates that most minor food sensitivities and allergies are resolved by correcting hypothyroidism and nutritional imbalances.

If you have sensitivities that persist after following my program, you must begin to look for those groups of foods to which you react. Here are a few courses which you might wish to follow: (1) See a clinical ecologist—a physician who specializes in treating food allergy problems. If there are no clinical ecologists in your immediate area, read such books as *Dr. Mandell's 5-Day Food Allergy Relief System*, which will give you step-by-step instructions to test foods by means of an "elimination diet." Once aware of the foods to which you are sensitive, you can rotate them, eating none of the offending ones any more than once every four days.

22. Relax and enjoy your program. With time and persistence, you will take off or keep off excess weight which can contribute to a host of ailments, among them cardiovascular disorders, which are the subject of the next chapter.

12

HOW TO PREVENT A
HEART ATTACK—YOUR OWN!

*H*idden in the throats of unsuspecting millions is the reason for many—if not most—heart attacks: a subnormal
thyroid gland.

Unfortunately, establishment medical doctors still do not recognize this fact and instead continue to advocate avoidance of
many wholesome, nourishing cholesterol-containing foods for
the purpose of diminishing cardiovascular ailments. It is difficult to understand how they can overlook a mountain of evidence that hypothyroidism is a major silent assassin—a mountain
whose base was formed in England more than a century ago.

It all began with a case mentioned earlier—Dr. William M.
Ord's severely atherosclerotic female patient with the grossly
enlarged, fibrous, non-working thyroid gland; mucin-logged,

swollen tissues; and a tight-skinned, masklike face. Reports of similar cases by other contemporary doctors made the medical community aware that this new ailment was widespread and required special study. In 1883 the London Clinical Society formed a task force, including elite Harley Street physicians, for this purpose. In the course of five years, the medical researchers identified and investigated one hundred cases of myxedema.

Results of experiments, observations of patients and examinations of autopsies, reported in a hefty 300-page volume, revealed unequivocally that myxedema was caused by decreased function of the thyroid gland. Atherosclerosis, commonly found in these cases, received no more attention than other symptoms, inasmuch as cardiovascular ailments were a rarity then. Epidemics of contagious diseases finished off most people before they could live long enough to develop cardiovascular disease.

Then, in 1890, Viennese pathologists discovered that thyroid deficiency helps bring on heart attacks, thanks to the wisdom and foresight which Austrian Empress Maria Theresa had demonstrated some 100 years earlier. The Empress had passed a national law making it mandatory that the body of each patient who had died in a hospital go through the autopsy procedure. This law actually turned Austrian hospitals into laboratories of learning so that, in a real sense, Maria Theresa accelerated medical progress for the world.

Unfortunately, knowledge of heart attack prevention seemed of little value in the 1890s, because heart attacks were still uncommon. An idea had been born before its time—a solution for which there was no problem.

Yet for the sake of science, researchers pursued further experiments. They found that after the thyroid was removed from test animals, they always developed atherosclerosis and mucinlogged tissues. Next, Professor Kocher of Berne, Switzerland, a surgeon in a known goiter belt, found that after life-saving thyroidectomy in 101 human beings, the same thing happened. If he had not operated on them, however, their massive goiters would have compressed the windpipe and caused suffocation.

Professor Kocher's surgery proved to be only a delaying action, because the patients quickly developed atherosclerosis and other symptoms identical to those in Dr. Ord's classic case and soon died. To assure continued thyroid hormone production and save lives, Professor Kocher then developed a surgical technique for removing only the part of the thyroid gland threatening the windpipe.

During the same period, Professor T. Billroth, Vienna's most eminent surgeon, noted for perfecting the stomach ulcer operation still in use, totally removed gigantic goiters and, like Kocher, lost the lives he was trying to save.

Over and over, Austrian pathologists observed and reported that thyroidectomy invariably brought on exaggerated hardening of the arteries. Despite articles on the findings of Drs. Kocher and Billroth in the world's medical journals, surgeons in some enlightened nations persisted in their practice of total thyroid removal until the 1950s.

Intrigued by the devastating results of thyroidectomy, Dr. Billroth assigned his most brilliant student, von Eilsberg, to make further investigations of arterial changes in animals—sheep and goats—after removal of the thyroid gland. In 1895 von Eilsberg reported that thyroidectomy brought on all the symptoms of myxedema, including gross degeneration of arteries throughout the body. It is of great significance that the coronary arteries, which supply the heart with blood, nourishment and oxygen, were among those that underwent degeneration. Several years later, Drs. E. P. Pick and F. Pineless, also of Vienna, confirmed these findings but, in using fresh thyroid extract on subjects, were able to prevent premature damage to the arteries.

Supplementation with thyroid only appeared to be new at that time. Chinese doctors 2,000 years before Christ rejuvenated aging patients with failing faculties by means of an animal thyroid soup, with the result that patients felt younger, had more energy, and often regained ability to think and remember. Many centuries later, during Queen Victoria's reign, London's most prominent Harley Street doctors took a cue from the Chinese and served elderly and failing patients special sandwiches whose main ingredient was raw animal thyroid gland.

Many patients were squeamish about eating raw thyroid gland, so doctors looked for alternatives. One effort that failed was transplanting thyroid glands from the newly dead or from animals into hypothyroid patients. The body rejected this foreign tissue. Finally, after long and arduous experimentation, G. R. Murray, a British medical doctor, concocted a glycerine extract of fresh thyroid tissue, injecting the juice into patients. Although it achieved desired results, Dr. Murray found that his preparation rapidly oxidized and molded. Then he struck upon the idea of removing fat from the fresh animal glands and drying them. This process preserved the active thyroid principle.

Now he needed a patient to try his desiccated thyroid. A middle-aged woman with acute myxedema, not many heartbeats from death, volunteered. She never regretted her decision, because her symptoms disappeared, and she remained in excellent health for nineteen years, when she died of natural causes at seventy-two. Several times she stopped taking thyroid supplements and, in each instance, her former symptoms returned until she renewed her thyroid regime.

Although Dr. Murray's natural desiccated thyroid formula is still used—it has been improved upon through the years—much research on its importance in the prevention and cure of cardiovascular ailments has been forgotten. The result is millions of premature deaths. Revealing research reports on thyroid therapy now gather dust in the clamor for some new miracle cure for cardiovascular ailments, some new solution to an already solved problem.

To paraphrase someone wiser than I am, those who don't know medical history and fail to familiarize themselves with it are doomed to repeat it. But when will they become enlightened? How many years or decades from now? How many unnecessary deaths from now?

Today, for better or for worse, physicians are married to the dubious theory that a diet low in cholesterol and saturated fat will reduce serum cholesterol level and the hazards of serious cardiovascular ailments. Even in these days of instant divorce, doctors cannot make a public break from this spouse without losing face. Face saving seems more important than the truth.

In January, 1984, results of a ten-year, $150 million study of cholesterol by the National Institutes of Health (NIH) were announced. The major conclusions of the research were: (1) that there is a direct link between the level of blood serum cholesterol and heart disease; (2) that lowering cholesterol significantly reduces the incidence of heart disease; and (3) that in instances of marked elevation of cholesterol, use of the drug cholestyramine can significantly reduce coronary heart disease.

The fanfare that accompanied the NIH announcement was so loud that it drowned out many facts relevant to the case. Basil Rifkind, director of the study, stated that the NIH research strongly indicated that the more we lower dietary cholesterol and fat, the more we reduce the risk of heart attacks.

But Rockefeller University's Dr. Edward Ahrens, who has conducted cholesterol research for almost forty years, believes just the opposite. More concerned with factuality than diplomacy, he told *Time* magazine: "Since this was basically a drug study, we can conclude nothing about diet; such extrapolation is unwarranted, unscientific and wishful thinking."[1]

Few Americans are afflicted with severe familial hypercholesterolemia—super-high levels of blood cholesterol (just one in 500 suffers from even a moderate form of this disease, says the same issue of *Time*)—so Dr. Ahrens offers a second objection to the study: the anti-meat, butter and egg propaganda accompanying the NIH announcement. He says that denying everyone red meat, eggs and dairy products, when only a minute fraction of the population is afflicted with hypercholesterolemia, is reducing the joy of life unnecessarily.

Dr. John Story, Purdue University cardiologist, scoffs at what he calls "cholesterolphobia." In the same issue of *Time*, he indicates that we should not treat everyone with diet, just as we wouldn't give insulin to everyone for fear of their developing diabetes.

Dr. Michael F. Oliver, president of the British Cardiac Society and Duke of Edinburgh Professor of Cardiology, Edinburgh University, expressed a similar thought in *Modern Medicine*.[2] He feels that persons with very high cholesterol levels—265 mg/dl or greater—should be identified and assisted in lowering blood cholesterol. "This does not mean that the entire population should undergo a reduction in cholesterol levels," he states.

Quoted in the same issue, George V. Mann, M.D., associate professor of medicine and biochemistry at Vanderbilt University's School of Medicine, agrees that patients should be carefully screened for cholesterol levels, and those with a cholesterol level below 240 mg/dl should be "reassured that no specific treatment should be undertaken."

Dr. Mann, however, frowns on giving patients with high cholesterol levels the drug cholestyramine used in the NIH research project, since he feels that the drug presents problems. It is unpleasant to take, and 68 percent of subjects who took it in the NIH test experienced side effects, usually in the gastrointestinal tract. Professor Oliver admits to being disturbed about twenty-one cases of gastrointestinal cancer and eight deaths from this drug, as well as mouth and pharynx cancers.

In a letter of January 28, 1984, to the present authors, Edward R. Pinckney, M.D., coauthor with Cathey Pinckney of *The Cholesterol Controversy*, called attention to the hazard of using cholestyramine. Certainly there were fewer deaths in the group of men whose blood cholesterol was reduced with cholestyramine in relation to test subjects who did not take the drug: 37 out of 1,906, compared with 47 out of 1,900. Then he issued a king-sized caveat:

> There were 73 percent more gastrointestinal cancers and 800 percent more deaths from these cancers in the group that took the drug. This coincides with previously reported animal studies which showed that the drug cholestyramine is not absorbed from the intestine but remains active throughout the bowels and is a known promoter of colon cancer when a cancer-inducing agent is given with the drug. Who knows what food, drink or chemical can be cancer causing?
>
> Lowering of blood cholesterol in this way has also been reported to increase the incidence of gallstones. In this study, those taking the drug had a 45 percent increase in gallstones when compared with those not taking the drug. Forty-four percent more of the men taking the drug had to have gallstone-related surgery (with all of that operation's attendant risks).
>
> Other bile duct diseases were greater by 22 percent in the group taking the drug. And 170 percent more of the men taking the drug complained of heartburn.
>
> When deaths as a result of accident and/or violence were compared, there were 175 percent more of these deaths in the group taking the drug. These figures include 100 percent more suicides, 100 percent more homicides and 200 percent more accidents than in the group that did not take the drug.
>
> All the percentages were calculated in the same way as they were in the study employed to show benefits of the drug (reported in the *Journal of the American Medical Association*, January 20, 1984).

Are such risks worth the possible lessening of coronary heart disease by the reported 20.6 percent?

Other pertinent questions are equally troublesome. Why was $150 million spent on cholesterol research involving a drug whose negative effects outweigh the positive? And how did medical science ever get side-tracked with recommending avoidance of dietary cholesterol and saturated fat, a practice which fails to address the basic problem?

It all began in 1913 with the Russian physiologist N. Anitschkov, who drew an erroneous conclusion from one of the faultiest experiments ever designed by a scientist. To gain information of use to human beings, the experimenter usually selects a member of the animal kingdom whose physiological processes closely resemble those of human beings.

Anitschkov's history-changing work revolved around rabbits fed huge doses of cholesterol. Rabbits are vegetarians. No self-respecting rabbits would ever eat cholesterol-containing foods. Their livers are not equipped to handle them chemically. As a result of this unnatural diet, the cholesterol content of their blood skyrocketed by several hundred percent and, in the end, these high concentrations of cholesterol proved toxic to them. This severe biochemical stress caused some atherosclerosis and the appearance of cholesterol in arterial lesions. To Anitschkov's credit, he realized that his research results did not necessarily apply to human beings, and he never suggested a low-cholesterol diet to control atherosclerosis.

Many decades later, in 1964, an explanation of the rabbit findings emerged from Anitschkov's laboratory through one of his proteges, L. V. Malysheva, who, in a published paper, reported that huge doses of cholesterol suppressed rabbit thyroid function as thoroughly as surgical removal of the thyroid gland.[3]

However subnormal thyroid function comes about, the result is the same: the development of atherosclerosis. Malysheva explained that deteriorated arteries in the rabbits were due to low thyroid function, not to cholesterol itself.

Researchers in Anitschkov's lab, Malysheva included, rejected the cholesterol theory, and American physicians embraced it.

Another biochemist, I. B. Friedland, a student of Anitschkov's, did much research on cholesterol and fats and in 1933 published a comprehensive report, representing five years of study. He made a significant discovery. When he fed rabbits large amounts of cholesterol, as Anitschkov had done, he was able to prevent the development of high levels of blood cholesterol and atherosclerosis by administering thyroid hormone to them. He concluded that thyroid hormone controls blood fat and cholesterol levels and recommended thyroid therapy in human beings with elevated fats in the blood serum.[4]

Dr. Barnes once told me that "if the Friedland recommendation had been followed, cardiovascular diseases would have been conquered decades ago and much time and many lives would have been saved."

In the cholesterol controversy, a key question is whether this fatty substance plays a major role in the deterioration of arteries. More than 125 years ago, Rudolph Virchow, professor of pathology and the father of what was then a new science, performed many autopsies and concluded that cholesterol has only a minor influence. In a paper published in Berlin, he revealed that degeneration of the blood vessels' connective tissue had started before cholesterol appeared in the lesions. Next, drops of fat accumulated there and then, finally, came cholesterol. Virchow considered cholesterol a belated sign of fatty degeneration.[5]

Another research finding that deflated the cholesterol balloon was that of a German physician, H. Zondek, during World War I.[6] With Germany isolated from the rest of the world and supplies of protein foods running low, military personnel as well as civilians were, of necessity, eating mainly grains and vegetables—a low-cholesterol, low-fat diet.

Dr. Zondek, who was in charge of a ward of cardiac patients, made the astute observation that these soldiers had all the symptoms of myxedema, the most dominant of which was heart failure. The usual treatment for heart disorders at that time was digitalis, which had already failed to help his other patients, many of whom were bed-ridden. Inasmuch as they had swollen tissues, no energy, shortness of breath and enlarged hearts, he decided to try thyroid therapy. Much to his surprise and delight, his patients were soon able to return to military duty or civilian life. He gave the name "myxedema heart" to their former ailment.

Soon after the war, Dr. Zondek wrote *Diseases of the Endo-*

crine Glands, a book translated into English in 1944, featuring illustrations of electrocardiograms of some of his patients. Individuals with "myxedema heart" showed low voltage, because of weak heartbeats. After thyroid therapy, when the heart contracted with more power, the voltage on the EKG returned to normal. A low voltage reading on the EKG reveals the status of the thyroid gland more accurately than many common blood tests for thyroid function, as many doctors have discovered.

Have we been unduly alarmed about intake of cholesterol in relation to blood serum levels of this compound? Numerous studies in various nations indicate that we have.

The much-publicized fourteen-year Framingham study of thousands of individuals, aimed at revealing the major risk factors for heart attack, failed to zero in on dietary cholesterol as the enemy within, despite the pre-study assertion by Dr. William B. Kannel, the project's director, that the blood test for cholesterol levels was perhaps the most useful method for determining present or impending heart disease. Results of the study changed his opinion.[7] Half the people who died of heart attacks failed to show the high cholesterol levels he believed warned of impending danger.

As a matter of fact, Dr. Kannel saw "no discernable association between the amount of cholesterol in the diet and the level of cholesterol in the blood." Regardless of how much or how little animal fat is in the diet, some people will have low blood cholesterol levels, while others will have moderate levels and others high levels, he stated.

Not long ago, the University of California School of Medicine fed 1,934 men and women anywhere from zero to fourteen eggs each week. Although one large egg contains about 250 mg of cholesterol, researchers were surprised to find no statistically significant relationship between number of eggs consumed and the blood serum cholesterol level.

Some years earlier, experimenters at the University of California at Los Angeles under Dr. Roslyn Alfin-Slater found no increase in cholesterol levels on normal diets when egg intake was increased.[8]

"We, like everyone else, had been convinced that when you eat cholesterol, you get cholesterol," she told the *Los Angeles Times*. "But when we stopped to think that all the studies in the past never tested the normal diet in relation to egg eating ... we decided to see what happened to blood cholesterol levels on normal diets when egg intake was increased. Our finding surprised us...."

The research of Professor A. H. Ismail at Purdue University confirmed the results of the UCLA group.[9]

Eggs are not really saboteurs of health. Researchers at Massachusetts Institute of Technology found that by eating two eggs per day, subjects benefited from the 5 grams of lecithin in the yolks.[10] They learned that within twenty-one days, such a regime increased the brain's plasma choline content by 500 percent, enhancing the synthesis of acetycholine, a key neurotransmitter of the brain. Results of this study indicate that lecithin can be helpful in restoring short-term memory loss.

Does a high-polyunsaturated-fat diet actually prevent or cure cardiovascular ailments? A six-year study in England is typical of research undertaken to establish the facts.[11] Four hundred elderly men were divided into two groups. Half of them were fed a diet high in polyunsaturated fats—no less than three ounces of polyunsaturated oil daily, plus polyunsaturated margarine. Whole milk, butter, cheese, egg yolks and saturated cooking fats were forbidden. The other half stayed on their usual diet, which contained six times as much saturated fat as polyunsaturated fat.

At first, cholesterol levels came down in the first group, a common occurrence with this sort of diet. Then, after the initial year, they began to rise. Following conclusion of the study, the cholesterol levels of the first group were about the same as when they started. Blood cholesterol of the saturated-fat eaters stayed virtually the same, too. However, the death rate from cardiovascular disease was slightly higher in the group which ate polyunsaturates—27 patients to 25. Results of a study conducted in Oslo, Norway, under similar conditions, were almost the same.

If the low-cholesterol diet is so effective, how can one account for the results of the Roseto, Pennsylvania, study, reported in the *Journal of the American Medical Association*, and studies of Somali camel herdsmen, the Masai tribe of Taganyika, and natives of the Cook Islands?[12]

Citizens of Roseto eat a diet that sounds like a shortcut to suicide to low-cholesterol advocates—all of the "no-no's": eggs, fatty meat, foods fried in lard, and other high-cholesterol delicacies such as prosciutto ham, rimmed by half an inch to an inch of saturated fat, and peppers fried in lard. But their blood cholesterol levels ranged from 136 to 500, averaging 224, comparable with that of participants in the Framingham study, about average for the nation. Shouldn't such an outrageous diet cause an abnormally high death rate from heart ailments? Let's look at the facts. After an eleven-year study, there were hardly any heart attacks in men under age fifty-five. In men over sixty-five who showed symptoms of heart disease, the rate of survival was high.

Somali camel herdsmen drink an average of five quarts of high-fat camel milk daily. Shouldn't their blood cholesterol level rocket out of sight? Actually, the highest blood serum cholesterol reading among them was 153. The Masai tribe lives almost entirely on meat and milk (whose fat content is almost twice that of ours) and shows a cholesterol level around 125 and negligible heart disease. Those over sixty-five autopsied after accidental death reveal only negligible signs of atherosclerosis. Comparisons have been made between two groups of Cook Islands Polynesians, one of which eats twelve times as much saturated fat as the other. Heart attacks were almost non-existent in both groups.[13]

Because some authorities claim that low-cholesterol diets work, and others claim the opposite and have statistics to back them, Drs. Stewart Wolf of the University of Texas and John Bruhn of the University of Oklahoma Medical School analyzed more than 100 articles from all over the world to isolate a dietary common denominator which might be considered a risk factor. They could find no consistent pattern about a certain kind of fat or a particular cholesterol level which seemed to cause heart disease.[14]

Another landmark study reveals some fascinating information about diet and heart disease, and that will be the subject of the next chapter.

13

BE KIND TO YOUR ARTERIES!

*O*ne of the prime arguments of those who favor the low-cholesterol diet is that heart attacks in Europe decreased drastically during World War II because of the scarcity of high-cholesterol foods.

Dr. Broda Barnes investigated this matter in depth, spending many summers in Graz, Austria, examining some of the world's most complete and definitive autopsy records.

"It is true that cholesterol-containing foods were scarce in Europe during World War II," he told me. "And, yes, heart attacks did decrease, but the interpretation of these facts led many investigators to the wrong conclusion. They failed to probe deeply enough. Instead of checking records of autopsies, they only counted the number of persons who had died of heart attacks."

So, in order to learn the truth for the protection of the living, Dr. Barnes went to the dead, checking 70,000 autopsies recorded between 1930 and 1970.

Heart attacks had dropped sharply in the war years between 1939 and 1945. But he discovered unexpected evidence that astonished him. *The low-fat diet had not protected arteries from atherosclerosis!* Autopsies revealed that the number of individuals under age fifty with atherosclerosis had doubled between 1939 and 1954. Further, the degree of injury to the arteries of these persons was approximately twice as great on a scale of zero to four. Not only had the low cholesterol diet failed to guard the arteries, but atherosclerosis had increased four-fold.

Why?

"We found that tuberculosis had risen far faster than heart attacks as the cause of death," said Dr. Barnes. "Tuberculosis victims rarely live beyond forty years—not quite long enough to have heart attacks.

"In most instances, those who died of tuberculosis showed extreme damage to coronary arteries. It is clear that if the adult patients had not died of tuberculosis, they would have been cut down by a heart attack in a short time. Wartime conditions had substituted tuberculosis for heart attacks as the major cause of death. Low-cholesterol diets had had nothing to do with protecting the people from heart attacks.

"A few years later, conditions were reversed," says Dr. Barnes. "The antibiotics for tuberculosis had become available, and deaths from heart attacks started to rise. The autopsies told us why: the adult dying from a heart attack had healing tuberculosis in his or her lungs. The antibiotics had stopped immediate death from tuberculosis, giving the advanced arterial damage a chance to become the killer."[1]

Dr. Barnes is not the only researcher who has found that the low-fat diet often fails to prevent heart attacks and that a high-fat diet does not necessarily bring on heart attacks. One of the most comprehensive projects, the Tecumseh study conducted by Allen B. Nichols, M.D., and his colleagues at the University of Michigan School of Medicine, reported similar findings and additional insight into causes for high serum cholesterol and triglycerides, a blood fat believed to contribute to cardiovascular ailments. The researchers checked almost the entire adult population of Tecumseh, Michigan, to determine the effect diet and overweight might have on blood cholesterol and triglyceride levels. The influence of 110 different food items—high or low in fats and sugar—on 4,057 persons was tabulated.

An article in the *Journal of the American Medical Association* (October 26, 1976) reported these findings: There was no significant relationship between how frequently fat, sugar, starch, alcohol and tea were consumed and the blood serum level of fats. Serum cholesterol and triglyceride concentrations were significantly higher in markedly overweight men and women. High fat levels in the bloodstream have long been associated with increased risk of heart disease and other health problems.

Dr. Nichols warns that these findings do not mean that diet and blood fat levels are not at all related, only that obesity more obviously raises serum cholesterol and triglyceride levels than any particular dietary regime.

"Other factors besides fat intake determine cholesterol levels among the general public," he says. "From this study's findings, one may infer that weight reduction should be the initial course for control of hyperlipidemia in the general population."[2]

Other studies indicate that more is involved in elevated cholesterol levels than intake of fats. Several researchers have found, for instance, that low thyroid function encourages high blood cholesterol. Experiments by the physiologist L. M. Hurxthal in the early 1930s revealed that blood cholesterol levels were high in hypothyroids and low in hyperthyroids.[3]

In their 1940 book, *The Biochemistry of Disease*, Bodansky and Bodansky went a step farther, stating that the rise in cholesterol in hypothyroidism is just a part of the total pattern of increased blood fats. They claimed a close relationship between appropriate thyroid supplementation and a decline in these symptoms.

The relationship between low thyroid function and high serum cholesterol level found by three researchers, E. F. Gildea, C. B. Mann and J. P. Peters, indicates that a serum cholesterol level below 275 mg percent practically excludes the diagnosis of hypothyroidism. Gildea discovered that two grains of thyroid would reduce cholesterol and triglyceride levels.

Bodansky and Bodansky make the interesting point that hypothyroidism can be diagnosed by high blood cholesterol, and effectiveness of treatment can be determined by the decline in blood serum level of cholesterol. A give-and-take relationship apparently exists between the decrease in basal metabolism in thyroid deficiency and the rise in blood cholesterol. *"On the average, the rise in cholesterol is approximately four times as great as the drop in metabolism."*[4] (Emphasis added.)

It remains a mystery to me why modern medicine fails to make use of this information. Perhaps it is because, during the mid-1930s, physicians started patients on too high dosages of thyroid and brought on heart attacks and, in several instances, death. The customary treatment for heart failure in that period was digitalis, administered in large dosages to saturate the patient, then in reduced dosages to maintenance level. No procedure could have been more wrong for thyroid. Large to massive dosages were tried—anywhere from 4 to 30 grains daily—causing the heart to race beyond its ability. From this flagrant misuse, thyroid developed a bad name, one it is still having difficulty overcoming. It is perhaps for this reason that a prime way to lower critical blood fats, including cholesterol, is often denied to patients who need it.

Like the word *thyroid*, the word *cholesterol* usually triggers a negative reaction—with little justification. Cholesterol is much denounced and disparaged in medical circles and a great deal of information and misinformation has been spread about this waxy, gray-yellow, fat-like alcohol which does not readily dissolve in water or blood. If we and the rest of the animal kingdom had no cholesterol, we would be part of the vegetable kingdom. (Vegetables contain no cholesterol.) Without a steady supply of this substance, we probably would not be around to complain about it. Cholesterol is so vital to our life that we have a built-in mechanism in the liver and in each body cell to manufacture it. Ideally, when cholesterol intake is high, the liver and cells gear down production. When intake is low, they increase production.

If you take in a great deal of dietary cholesterol, your body, if in proper balance, will get rid of the excess. The amount of cholesterol you eat, therefore, doesn't automatically have a real relationship to its level in your blood serum. If you literally stuff yourself on cholesterol-rich foods, the small intestine provides the built-in protection of limiting absorption. Excess cholesterol does not make it through the intestinal wall and into the bloodstream. It simply exits from the body through the bowel.

Contrary to the opinion of some, cholesterol can be synthesized from carbohydrates and proteins, as well as from fats. Therefore, no matter what kind of diet you eat, your body will have plenty of raw material to be made into cholesterol. If eaters of eggs, milk products and meat happen to have a slightly higher blood cholesterol level than vegetarians, the reason may be simple, says one observer. When animal fats are digested, they are not soluble in water or blood serum. Therefore, intestinal tract cells must synthesize cholesterol to unite with them so that they can be transported through the bloodstream to be metabolized or stored. It is this synthesized cholesterol—not dietary cholesterol—that may raise the blood serum level of animal fat eaters. Vegetable fats are more soluble in water and thus require less cholesterol to be produced in the intestinal tract to promote their utilization.

Why do we need cholesterol, anyway? For many reasons.

It is a *must* for the creation of a new life. When the sperm cells of a man join the egg of a woman to create a new human being, they bring along their own supply of cholesterol. In a short time the mother-to-be's blood serum level of cholesterol rises by about 50 percent, the liberal amount necessary to supply the cholesterol needed by the fetus's trillions of cells until birth. Dr. Broda Barnes makes the wry comment that if cholesterol were harmful to arteries, as so many have stated, "the fetus would have a heart attack before the baby saw the light of day."

The newborn baby comes fully equipped with the right enzymes to make possible the production of cholesterol in each cell, a necessity for the growth of tissue and for development of the brain. As adults, we no longer can synthesize cholesterol in the brain for a very good reason: we don't need to. Cholesterol already there and in the spinal cord—about 23 percent of the total in the body—is used and reused. Some authorities believe that brain cholesterol serves as part of the insulation for myriad nerve fibers there and as a non-conducting separator to prevent short-circuiting.

Cholesterol has other uses. It helps make fats soluble to be burned as fuel for muscles and connective tissue, the supporting members for various organs. About 10 percent of body cholesterol is in the skin, where it has a well-known use. Through a chemical reaction to sunlight, skin cholesterol produces vitamin D, which makes possible the assimilation of calcium and phosphorus essential to forming and sustaining strong bones and teeth. It also helps the growth of new skin to replace that which is scratched, cut or burned.

You may not be aware of the contribution cholesterol makes to your body in emergencies: it serves as the basic building blocks for hormones produced by the adrenal glands. Without cholesterol, you couldn't survive stress-filled situations.

Despite cholesterol's all-important role in the body, it is still regarded by many as the enemy within. But does eating high-cholesterol foods really elevate our serum cholesterol? Not necessarily. Individuals from families with a pronounced record of early heart disease have been shown to develop elevated cholesterol levels from a high-cholesterol diet. Other than that, the evidence that food intake causes this condition is inconclusive at best. Then what causes high blood cholesterol levels?

Heredity is probably a major contributing factor. Our anxiety and stress levels are also causes. Students before critical exams, athletes prior to key games, military men and women before combat (fliers, particularly) and accountants at tax time all have elevated cholesterol. High blood pressure, obesity, smoking, high blood uric acid levels, little or no exercise, and being male have all been associated with increased cholesterol levels.

One of the most dramatic and promising ways of reducing elevated cholesterol is, unfortunately, not as well known as it should be. It involves increasing the ratio of high density lipoproteins (HDL) to low density lipoproteins (LDL). If you have more HDL than LDL, your chances of escaping a heart attack are far more favorable.

Earlier we mentioned that fats and water don't mix well—usually not at all. The way that fats (including cholesterol) can be transported in the watery medium of the bloodstream is by becoming attached to lipoproteins, a combination of fat and protein. The best information today holds that LDL carries fats and cholesterol to the cells, including those in the arteries, and deposits them there. HDL units are like mini dump trucks that haul off excess cholesterol (some think they even remove cholesterol from cells) and carry it to the liver for elimination from the body.

There are five effective ways of increasing the ratio of HDL to LDL: (1) refrain from smoking; (2) exercise vigorously (check with your doctor first); (3) slash your intake of calories (become or stay fairly lean); (4) substitute some unsaturated fats (for instance, those in fish and fowl) for saturated; (5) eat certain foods and food supplements, such as cold-water fish, brewer's yeast, garlic and lecithin.[6]

Instant results are not guaranteed. The program must be pursued for a period, particularly if you are middle-aged or older.

Now, finally, through the HDL theory, scientists are beginning to understand what they have known for many years: that regular and vigorous exercise helps to prevent cardiovascular disease. A team of researchers led by Josef Patsch at Baylor College of Medicine found that jogging actually clears fats from the blood. Markedly higher levels of HDL were discovered in physically active individuals. How does this come about, according to the Patsch theory?

Within several hours after a meal, fat particles in the bloodstream (chylomicrons) encounter a blood enzyme which digests part of their cores. The remains are carried to the liver for digestion. Surfaces of the fat particles are then released by a blood enzyme and unite with other blood chemicals to become HDL.

Patsch does not understand exactly how exercise increases HDL. However, his research indicates that vigorous exercise must be continued regularly to keep HDL levels high. Such exercise must be pursued for at least several months to increase HDL to a pronounced degree, and it declines rapidly if one becomes inactive. In other words, quick-fix exercise is not going to help much. You have to exercise vigorously for a lifetime to extend your lifespan and improve your health. Eliminating high-fat and cholesterol-rich foods to lower blood fats and cholesterol will not do the trick. Such an approach does not take into consideration that health and illness are functions of many factors, not just a single unproven one.

Let's take a close look at how and why cholesterol affects the body.

Arteries are lifelines for channeling blood from the heart to living cells in constant need of nourishment and oxygen for burning their fuel. They must be kept clear, or trouble results.

A cross-section of human blood vessels reveals three layers of tissue. The innermost is an ingenious, smooth and slippery lining which permits near frictionless flow of blood. Enclosing the inner layer is a circle of muscle fibers which permits the blood vessels to expand and contract as the heart expands and contracts. On the outside is the third layer, coarse and stout connective tissue to reinforce the blood vessels or the arteries.

Blockages occur where there has been wear and tear on the artery wall. An irregular area is presumably the starting point for a buildup of cholesterol which, in time, can slow or stop the blood flow.

Some scientists speculate that arterial degeneration starts in the wall of the artery. Nature will not overlook such a defect, so she attempts to cope with it. Fibrin, a blood component essential to clotting, seals the stress point and begins a buildup on it. Pathologist Rudolph Virchow noted that this occurs long before cholesterol becomes involved. In performing autopsies he discovered that arterial deterioration started long before blood fat began to cling to the fibrin, and that this was followed by the accumulation of cholesterol. He also discovered that a person's circulation almost shut itself off before cholesterol attached itself to the plaque on the artery walls.

Numerous pathologists have since come to the same conclusion: cholesterol buildup in the wall of arteries occurs only after arterial degeneration is far advanced. It seems strange, then, that cholesterol is singled out when arterial plaque is composed not only of cholesterol but also of fibrin, calcium, triglycerides, ceroids and sometimes blood platelets.

Although numerous studies done long ago showed the thyroid connection in the degeneration of arteries, a striking study in more recent times demonstrates the value of thyroid therapy to the hearts and arteries of hypothyroid patients.

In a monograph, *Thyroid Function and Its Possible Role in Vascular Degeneration*, Dr. William B. Kountz reviewed earlier experiments linking low thyroid and deteriorating arteries and studied 288 hypothyroid patients with elevated blood cholesterol—his own and those at the infirmary of Washington University, St.

Louis. These included (1) businessmen averaging fifty-five years of age; (2) infirmary outpatients whose ages averaged sixty-one and (3) infirmary inpatients averaging sixty-seven years of age.[7]

Few in the first group had atherosclerosis. Many in the second group were found to have moderate cardiovascular degeneration. Everyone in the third group showed evidence of advanced blood vessel disease.

Dr. Kountz administered thyroid to some in each group and kept others as controls. After five years of observation, he compared those on thyroid therapy with controls on the basis of number of deaths from heart attacks and strokes.

In the first group—the youngest men—no one on thyroid therapy died, compared with 15 percent of the controls. Effects of thyroid treatment were most marked in the older men. Only 3 percent of the second group died, compared with 19 percent of the controls. In the third group, the fatality rate was half as high among those on thyroid as among the controls.

While assuring proper thyroid gland function or adequate supplementation seems the most basic approach to protecting or regaining a healthy cardiovascular system, sometimes other measures help, too, such as proper intake of vitamins, particularly vitamins C, B6 and E.

An article in *Lancet* stated that 1000 mg of vitamin C daily lowered cholesterol levels of healthy individuals and that long-term shortage of this vitamin contributed to arterial diseases which invite heart attacks and strokes.

Rabbit experiments conducted by Dr. Anthony Verlangieri of Rutgers University revealed that lack of vitamin C in the daily diet brought about the loss of certain chemical compounds in the artery linings, creating roughness and irregularities where harmful plaques could readily form. High blood levels of vitamin C increased the amount of these chemicals, helping assure that artery linings stay smooth.[8]

In an article in the *Journal of the American Geriatric Society*, Dr. M. L. Riccitelli of the Yale School of Medicine reported various experiments over twenty-two years which paralleled Dr. Verlangieri's findings.[9]

Several investigators have discovered that vitamin C-deprived animals developed atherosclerotic lesions like those in human beings and were cured by administration of vitamin C over long periods of time. Vitamin C not only reduced blood cholesterol levels but seemed to prevent cholesterol accumulation on artery linings.

Research done by Constance Spittle Leslie, M.D., a pathologist at Pinderfields Hospital in Wakefield, Yorkshire, England, convinced her that atherosclerosis is a deficiency disease similar to beriberi, scurvy, rickets and pellagra, caused by poor diet and reversible by corrective nutrition. Many of her findings have been published by the prestigious medical journal *Lancet.*

Dr. Leslie conducted an important experiment on herself. Noting that her cholesterol count dropped sharply when she ingested what are considered by some to be large doses of vitamin C, she reduced her cholesterol count from 230 to 140 by taking more liberal amounts of vitamin C. She then brought her cholesterol levels right up by restricting her vitamin C intake.[10]

Another vitamin, too, seems to influence cholesterol levels and atherosclerosis, vitamin B6. Dr. Roger Williams cites a Russian experiment which revealed low blood plasma levels of vitamin B6 in co-enzyme form in 31 of 48 patients with atherosclerosis and high cholesterol counts, and he theorizes that vitamin B6 contributes to body production of lecithin, a dissolver of cholesterol.[11] On the basis of this and other experiments, Dr. Williams advises that daily intake of sufficient vitamin B6 is one of the best guarantees against harm from fat and cholesterol combined with proteins.

Although many claims of early experimenters with vitamin E relative to cardiovascular ailments have not been substantiated, more recently this vitamin has been found to monitor and regulate magnesium and manganese penetration into heart cells, to enhance microcirculation and to reduce arterial deterioration in the legs.

One theory of how arteries deteriorate is that they are attacked at their weak points by free radicals, highly active atoms or molecules. Any irregular site invites deposits of fats, cholesterol and calcium. Vitamin E is a known killer of free radicals and, as such, protects the integrity of arteries. Vitamin E also normalizes clotting time of blood, minimizing or eliminating the chance of clots that can block arteries and take lives.

Additionally, vitamin E has a proven track record in managing intermittent claudication, leg pain caused by obstructed circulation. Probably the most impressive performance relative to this condition was revealed in a seven-year study by Sweden's Knut Haeger, M.D., a vascular surgeon.[12]

Those who suffer from intermittent claudication can walk only a short distance before the pain becomes unbearable. Once they stop walking, the pain slowly recedes. Dr. Haeger found that as little as 300 to 400 IU a day of vitamin E and daily walking brought about two results within several months: the ability of patients to walk longer distances before experiencing pain and increased blood circulation to the lower leg.

His 220 age-matched subjects (including some diabetics) had limited flow of blood to the feet. Such patients are subject to gangrene, a decaying of the flesh which follows choking off of the blood supply. The subjects were divided into two groups. Half received 300 IU of vitamin E daily; the other half were given placebos. During the seven-year period, only one of the patients on vitamin E had to have a leg amputated because of gangrene, compared with eleven on the placebo.

Dr. Haegar's experiment and those cited earlier offer convicing evidence that vitamins are valuable in efforts to manage vascular disorders.

It is customary to think of artery ailments in terms of extremes—gangrene, deadly heart attacks and strokes. Yet there is a whole range of illnesses in various parts of the body which arise from imperfect arteries—conditions which can be prevented and, in many instances, reversed, if the proper measures are taken. That is the subject of the next chapter.

14

DRAMATIC TREATMENT FOR
CIRCULATORY PROBLEMS

So far as circulatory ailments are concerned, headlines and millions of words are devoted to strokes and heart attacks, but little helpful information is offered about the prevention of less extreme yet still disabling complaints arising from chronic arterial disease.

The major disorders of this kind are neuropathies (nerve deterioration which often limits leg, arm or eye function), kidney failure, detached retina, blindness and—perhaps most frightening—gangrene. These often painful and handicapping conditions can limit the lifespan of anyone, particularly diabetics and the elderly. The good news is that something tangible can be done about these ailments.

As matters now stand, almost 98 percent of some 11 million

diabetics in the United States will suffer one or more of these complaints, the nightmarish complications of diabetes. Unfortunately, most of them do not know that with preventive health maintenance they can very likely be spared these health catastrophes.

A specific example will illustrate this point. At a party a number of years ago, I heard a woman say, "My eyesight is beginning to fail as a result of my diabetes, and my doctor tells me he can't do a thing about it." The dismal prospect offered this woman by her physican was just to wait around to go blind.

Turning abruptly, I said to her, "I just overheard your last remark. I'm a medical doctor and I may be able to help you."

I made an appointment for her to visit my office five days later, after she had taken her armpit temperature on two consecutive days.

Sure enough, she was hypothyroid. I put her on a grain of thyroid and, after a month, when her temperature had failed to move upward, increased it to two grains.

Within nine weeks, she was feeling better than she had since the age of twenty-five and, even more satisfying to her, her eyesight remained 20-40 without glasses. Even after five years her eyes still test 20-40. Not long ago when I saw her, she gave me an undeserved compliment.

"Doctor, I owe my eyesight to you."

"Thanks for the compliment," I responded. "I helped, but you actually owe your eyesight to Broda Barnes, a medical doctor who made the discovery concerning diabetic complications that I used in your case and in others."

As far as I am concerned, Dr. Barnes is worthy of a Nobel prize in medicine for many solid reasons, one of the most important of which is his discovery that thyroid supplementation in diabetics who are hypothyroids can stop diabetic complications and, in some instances, even reverse them. I know this is true from my own practice and from that of others who follow Dr. Barnes's methods.

In my opinion, Dr. Barnes's contribution is the most noteworthy breakthrough for diabetics since the discovery of insulin. It all began in 1965, when he suddenly realized that twelve diabetic patients whom he had treated for fifteen years showed no signs of diabetic complications.

Then came additional surprises.

His new diabetic patients with atherosclerosis, very high blood cholesterol levels, nerve deterioration and impaired eye or leg movement experienced what modern medicine thought impossible: an arresting of these conditions and, sometimes, reversals and complete cures. Over the next fifteen years, forty-three diabetic patients who came to him were put on thyroid supplementation, and none manifested the slightest sign of typical diabetic complications.

A clear picture began to emerge. Dr. Barnes went to the medical literature and soon learned that several other medical doctors had independently discovered what he had and had published papers on the subject in important medical journals. These illuminating, life-saving articles had been overlooked or ignored by most physicians and eventually forgotten.

Dr. Barnes was appalled. In the years between the publication of these articles and 1965, hundreds of thousands—even millions—of diabetics had unnecessarily gone through pain, disability, depression and early death.

Among significant studies yellowing in medical libraries was the 1930 research of Dr. Elliott P. Joslin, founder of Boston's Joslin Clinic. Before Drs. Banting and Best had extracted a safe and effective preparation of insulin in 1921, diabetics usually lived only four years after their illness was diagnosed. Now their lifespan was extended. Instead of dying in a coma, diabetics were living seven years longer and then dying of different causes, among them heart attacks. Insulin was unable to prevent these devastating complications.

One of the few persons to understand the basic reasons for complications of diabetics, Dr. Joslin published his findings in the best medical journals and predicted that some day atherosclerosis would be conquered and that subsequently the diabetic would live a normal lifespan.

Most diabetologists snubbed his findings and the heretical notion that insulin was not the final solution. They maintained that all physicians had to do was diagnose diabetes early enough and treat it vigorously enough.

"So they diagnosed it early and treated it vigorously, and, judging from their results, not early or vigorously enough," according to Dr. Barnes. Because of the longer life of diabetics, more complications of this ailment had time to appear. Foremost among them was hardening of the arteries.

"Even today, I find articles and books making the nonsensical statement that diabetes aggravates or accelerates hardening of the arteries," snorts Dr. Barnes. "No way! Hypothyroidism is perhaps the leading cause of this condition."

In Dr. Barnes's nearly half a century as a general practitioner, none of his 5,000 patients (either with a normal thyroid gland or on thyroid hormone) has shown a sign of diabetic complications. Further, only five of his patients developed diabetes in this period. The national average is 200 per 5,000 individuals—*forty times higher.*

On two occasions, Dr. Barnes told me something that I have subsequently observed in my practice, namely, that the same kinds of complications observed in the diabetic also appear in the low thyroid patient and that, when thyroid is administered, some of these complications, particularly neuropathies, disappear.

All diabetic and hypothyroid complications arise from the same basic cause: clogged arteries which prevent the blood from bringing in food and oxygen and carrying off wastes.

Let's look at all the complications, starting with kidney failure. Kidney function is lost. Toxic wastes cannot be eliminated in the urine and accumulate in the bloodstream. Unless dialysis comes to the rescue, the patient dies of uremia.

A less common but even more devastating result of diabetic arteriosclerosis is gangrene. Gangrene occurs mainly in the legs, because their circulation is less efficient. The blood has to be forced against gravity back to the heart. In the fingers or arms, blood flows to the heart more easily.

Gangrene became much more prevalent after the discovery of insulin. Before this time, people generally did not live long enough to develop it. As critical as this condition is—and as difficult to treat—some patients have been spared the agony of developing it, thanks to Dr. Barnes's methods.

A new patient was brought to Dr. Barnes for treatment, a grey-haired sixty-year-old man who was paralyzed on one side from a recent stroke. As Walter lay on the examination table, a remote part of his anatomy caught Dr. Barnes's attention—the big toe of the right foot. It looked abnormally red and misshapen, like a moderate-size, rotten, mashed tomato. The paralysis and stroke suddenly became less important. Walter had gangrene! His poor circulation had been worsened because of his paralyzed side.

"Many a knife-happy surgeon would have lopped off that big toe," Dr. Barnes informed me, "but that wouldn't have stopped the gangrene. It keeps climbing to the ankles, then the thigh. Then it usually goes to the other side and starts all over. The knife fights a delaying action—at the end of the toe, then at the ankle, at the knee and finally at the thigh. The surgeon's knife operates the patient into disability and then, often, into death."

Dr. Barnes had an alternative. Gangrene and the stroke already told him that the patient had circulatory problems, perhaps of low thyroid origin. Learning that Walter had lived most of his life in the state of Indiana, a part of the great United States goiter belt, he had additional evidence of possible hypothyroidism. The underarm temperature test showed a subnormal reading of 96 degrees, just the confirmation Dr. Barnes needed. He administered one-half grain of desiccated thyroid per day and kept a close watch on the patient. Things happened fast. Within a week, the rotten, mashed tomato appearance of Walter's right big toe began changing. A month later, the toe was completely healed.

Remarkable recoveries from diabetic complications such as this encouraged Dr. Barnes to share his discoveries with other doctors. But a giant roadblock kept the mass of the medical community from even trying his method: the lack of controlled double-blind studies to prove his findings on a completely objective level.

"Rarely can a physician in private practice conduct controlled experiments," Dr. Barnes readily admits, "but he sometimes makes pertinent observations that deserve the attention of clinical investigators with facilities to give them further evaluation." Deserving attention and getting it were two different things.

Dr. Barnes has also had fascinating experiences in reversing neuropathies, which run the gamut from annoying to devastating. If atherosclerosis damages a nerve to the eye muscle, the patient may lose his or her ability to move the eye from side to side. Deterioration of nerves in the leg could make walking difficult or impossible.

One case which Dr. Barnes described in an interview is an

example of positive accomplishments which are possible with the thyroid treatment of neuropathies. A patient was referred to him by an Arizona doctor. Muscles between the man's left knee and thigh had become atrophied and weak. In excruciating pain, the patient had to take pain-killers day and night. He could hobble around for short distances but only with a cane.

The man was frustrated and depressed that his pain limited his daily activities and brought him agony. After verifying that this patient was hypothyroid, Dr. Barnes explained that he was going to put him on a small daily dosage of thyroid. Skeptical but willing to try anything, the patient agreed to take the thyroid but insisted on staying in a Fort Collins, Colorado, motel near Dr. Barnes's offices in the event that thyroid did not agree with him. (He had heard some of the ancient thyroid scare stories.)

Within one week, he was able to cut down on the pain-killer. His general health improvement encouraged him to go back to Arizona and continue thyroid supplementation. Within a month, he could walk painlessly without the cane and threw it away. Two years later—the last information Dr. Barnes had on the patient—his leg was completely normal.

Although some doctors still say that neuropathies in the eyes, which contribute to blindness, are caused by diabetes, this is not true. Atherosclerosis is the cause—deterioration of the tiny arteries of the eyes.

Although most doctors who have used thyroid hormone have been able to treat diabetics to prevent disabling neuropathies and blindness, perhaps the most dramatic and revealing work has been done by Drs. Michael Walczak of Studio City, California, Murray Israel of New York City, and I. R. Ross of Maryland, all members of the Vascular Research Foundation.[1]

Their findings add a ray of hope to the otherwise ominous information of the National Society for the Prevention of Blindness, which projects that some 50 percent of persons who have diabetes for at least twenty years will develop retinopathy (deterioration of the retina of the eye) while 95 percent of those who have diabetes for thirty years will probably develop this disease.

Drs. Walczak, Israel and Ross treat impending blindness (diabetic retinopathy) with oral thyroid hormone extract, heavy intakes of vitamin B complex, vitamin C and the natural enzyme varidase. Diuretics are also given to remove excess body fluid. Forty out of forty-five patients—twenty-five of whom were legally blind—were measurably improved after thirteen months on the above regime. Two did not improve, and three became worse. Such startling results came in the wake of a Harvard School of Public Health announcement that no cure exists for the progressively disabling complications of diabetes.

One of the most dramatic changes came in a patient who had been totally blind in one eye prior to taking part in the research project. Vision in his other eye was diminishing so fast—20/200—that he became almost a vegetable and sat around in a deep depression. Elevated cholesterol and blood pressure as well as irregularities of metabolism made him seem a prime candidate for failure in the project.

However, after five months on the Walczak-Israel-Ross regime, his blood pressure went down markedly, and his cholesterol reading plummeted from 294 to 215. Best of all, his vision improved to 20/60, and he became encouraged, recharged with optimism, more energetic, healthier and able to work again.

One of Dr. Walczak's patients experienced an equally exciting transformation, a forty-seven-year-old woman who was weak, had pain, cold extremities, albumen in the urine, advanced diabetic retinopathy, and was in a pre-gangrenous state. She came into the experiment with little hope, inasmuch as all other known treatment for retinopathy had done her no good. She was in such poor shape that Dr. Walczak wondered if she would live long enough to go blind.

On the thyroid-vitamins-enzyme-diuretic regime, she soon reported less pain, greater warmth in her extremities, more strength and endurance and no albumen in her urine. Rather than risk subjectivity, Dr. Walczak sent her to an impartial ophthalmologist for comparative measurement of her vision. In the words of this doctor, her progress was "almost unbelievable."

Still another of Dr. Walczak's cases, a sixty-six-year-old woman, had such deteriorating eyesight that she could see only foggy outlines of objects. A year after she joined the experiment, she could distinguish different flowers in pots twenty feet away. Then, five months later, came an incredible improvement. For the first time in years, she could read the newspaper. The independent and impartial ophthalmologist who tested her eyes found that her right eye had improved to 20/25 and the left to 20/40. Improvement continued.

Dr. Walczak believes that, effective as this form of treatment is even in what appear to be almost impossible cases, it is even better when used preventively, in the early stages of retinopathy, when the disease has not as yet begun to hamper vision. Eleven of twelve patients with retinal deterioration showed definite and encouraging improvement on this regime in one experiment.[2] While conservative physicians may want to wait for the results of double-blind studies before adopting this regime, every week, month, or year that passes may be critical to those with retinopathies and other complications of diabetes. There is no time for fence-sitting. Millions desperately need helpful treatment such as this. There is little time to waste with these patients before beginning thyroid therapy. It is time for those with sight and foresight to help those who are about to lose their sight and possibly their lives.

Unquestionably, much can be done to prevent arterial deterioration, as well as other diseases, including cancer, which is the one most feared by the most people. This is the subject of the next chapter.

15

GUARD YOURSELF
AGAINST CANCER

That tiny thyroid gland—less than an ounce in weight—can bring you pounds of prevention against cancer, a disease that picks its victims indiscriminately.

Interesting evidence links hypothyroidism and cancer. A survey by Dr. J. G. C. Spencer of Frenahay Hospital in Bristol, England, revealed a higher than average cancer rate in the goiter belts of fifteen nations on four continents.[1]

Subnormal thyroid function appears to invite cancer. This has been shown clinically in numerous animal experiments. Malignant tissue from rats grafted onto other rats took hold readily in those animals whose thyroid glands had been removed, but rarely in those with normal thyroid function.

Findings with thousands of laboratory rats as well as with

human beings by Dr. Bernard Eskin, director of endocrinology in the Department of Obstetrics and Gynecology at the Medical College of Philadelphia, indicate that a deficiency of iodine, one of the thyroid gland's major nutritional components, encourages breast cancer.[2] Dr. Eskin discovered that the highest incidence of breast cancer and deaths from it are in the goiter belts of Poland, Switzerland, Austria and the United States. The iodine-impoverished Great Lakes region of the coast-to-coast goiter belt shows the highest death rate from breast cancer in the United States. Conversely, iodine-rich Japan and Iceland have the world's lowest rates of goiter and deaths from breast cancer. In fact, the breast cancer death rate in Japan, where iodine-rich seafood and seaweed are on the daily menu, is one-fifth that of the United States.

As stated earlier, sufficient dietary iodine does not always assure proper thyroid gland function. However, normal function of this gland—or supplementation with thyroid extract—seems to deter cancer.

Studies show that hypothyroids and hyperthyroids appear to be more cancer-prone than the general population. Several years ago, there were the makings of a bitter controversy in this area. One faction named hypothyroidism a major cause. Other factions disagreed violently.

A German medical journal (*Klinical-Wochenshr.*) several years ago ran an article admitting that there is a keen difference of opinion among experts.[3] According to the authors, one group feels that a shortage of circulating thyroid hormones makes the skin of the breasts hypersensitive to prolactin (the pituitary gland hormone that promotes milk production) and estrogen. This could contribute to cancerous growths. But they also say that thyroid hormone replacement is associated with the risk of breast cancer. Other evidence disputes this stand, and the American Thyroid Association favors hypothyroid patients' continuing thyroid therapy, if such therapy is indicated.

As far as hyperthyroidism is concerned, the authors state that excess thyroid hormones in the blood seemed to slow the growth of inoperable breast cancer. This is disputed, too, they say, and refer to other findings which relate hyperthyroidism to the development of breast cancer in premenopausal women.

A subsequent report in the journal *Cancer* concluded that "a proportion of breast cancer patients are mildly hypothyroid...."[4] A year later, the *Journal of the American Medical Association* presented research by a team of eleven authorities, who conducted a case-control study to establish, once and for all, whether or not thyroid hormone therapy increases the risk of breast cancer.[5] The team compared 659 women with breast cancer and 1,719 control subjects and found no evidence that thyroid supplements increased the risk of breast cancer, even when thyroid supplements had been taken for more than fifteen years.

Thyroid replacement in hypothyroidism has been said to reverse cancer in some instances. One such case was presented in the journal *Neurology*.[6] A hypothyroid patient with a large tumor of the pituitary gland was given thyroid hormone. The tumor rapidly disappeared. Another case of a slightly different nature appeared in the *Southern Medical Journal.*[7] A woman with primary hypothyroidism was found to have a large pituitary tumor and, concurrently, the cessation of menstruation and an excessive flow of milk. Nine months after thyroid therapy was started, there was clinical and radiologic evidence that the tumor had regressed, along with the other symptoms.

These cases and the remarkable findings of John A. Myers, M.D., F.R.S.H., indicate that alternatives should be carefully examined before women patients are rushed into surgery, particularly for removal of the ovaries.[8]

Dr. Myers's success in treating serious female conditions by nonsurgical methods has opened new vistas for all physicians and their patients. It is Dr. Myers's opinion that, although cancer is a formidable enemy, we should not let cancer phobia run away with rational decision-making. The primitive fear of the unknown and the potent drive for survival sometimes stampede us into undesirable treatment alternatives. An atmosphere heavy with fear impels the surgeon who removes a cancerous breast to perform surgery on a normal, though susceptible, second breast. Occasionally, patients request this as a security measure. Likewise, when a cancerous uterus is removed, sometimes a sound ovary is cut out, too, for fear that cancer will develop there. On occasion, both ovaries are taken out.

Preventive surgery of the ovaries is easier to rationalize in women beyond menopause, as Dr. Myers indicates. The ovaries produce the hormones estrogen and progesterone, as well as ova. The first two can be replaced. So why not part with the ovaries? For a very good reason. The ovaries make another important and little-known contribution to survival and wellbeing, as Dr. Myers learned while reviewing a paper on atherosclerosis by Joseph Stambul, M.D., chief cardiologist, Department of Medicine, Southern Division of the Albert Einstein Medical Center.

Dr. Stambul stated that atherosclerosis in the coronary artery is six times more prevalent in men than in women, a key reason why women live longer than men. The obvious explanation—and a gross simplification—is that women produce estrogen. However, he also said that another hormone-like substance is synthesized by the ovaries—protein-bound iodine, or diiodotyrosine—which keeps cholesterol in solution in the blood, rather than allowing it to accumulate in the lining of arteries.

Long before he learned of Dr. Stambul's thesis, Dr. Myers claims that he had used diiodotyrosine to soften the breasts of nursing women, particularly hypothyroid women. He states correctly that cysts and abscesses can develop in breasts which become caked in nursing mothers and offers an example of a patient who had a hardened and painful left breast. He administered 200 grams of diiodotyrosine and, within two days, brought the breast back to good health. In another similar case, the mother's breasts were so painful and hard that they yielded too little milk to satisfy the baby. Over a period of several hours, the mother was given 10 grams of diiodotyrosine to dissolve under her tongue. Almost immediately her breasts softened, the pain ceased and milk began spurting from the nipples. That was the end of her nursing problems.

Still another female ailment was solved by the same method. A forty-five-year-old woman had a large abscess on her left breast and a cyst four millimeters long on her left ovary. The knowledgeable gynecologist who made the diagnosis recommended surgery for both conditions. Deeply upset, the woman appealed to Dr. Myers for treatment without surgery. Over a two-day period, he gave her some 50 grams of powdered diiodotyrosine to dissolve under her tongue, in addition to intravenous magnesium, B complex and vitamin C. Response came quickly: the ovarian cyst ruptured and the breast abscess came to a great head and spewed forth a good deal of pus. Both conditions healed rapidly. Inasmuch as the breasts were still quite hard, heavy and doughy, Dr. Myers continued the treatment. Within a matter of days, the breasts softened and regained the normal feeling of fluidity.

These are not isolated cases. Dr. Myers has had the same results in innumerable similar cases. He also tells of subduing persistent vaginal infections—trichomonas and yeast infection as well as nonspecific leukorrhea, which had resisted various treatments—in patients, most of whom were hypothyroid. Dr. Myers treated these patients with thyroid hormone and intra-vaginal iodine. Their hypothyroid condition cleared up and so did their infections. Within minutes after the vaginal treatment with iodine, several of the women with hardened breasts felt and saw a softening. Women with cysts had them disappear in time.

Such measures help ward off conditions which, in some instances, may be forerunners of cancer. Dr. Myers has validated the Stambul findings concerning the ovaries and the importance of their secretions in numerous cases, including the following:

Several weeks after her ovaries were surgically removed, a forty-six-year-old-woman found goiters swelling her throat. The woman, a Navy nurse, had had a total hysterectomy, including removal of her ovaries, in the Navy Hospital in Bethesda, Maryland. While recovering from her operation, she was found to have developed nodules on her thyroid gland. Alerted to the possibility of cancer, she was told to have the nodules removed. Rather than endure more surgery, she asked Dr. Myers to treat her. He did so with estrogen, iodine, vitamins and minerals. The thyroid nodules began shrinking slowly. After two years, they disappeared. Two years later when she was examined by Navy doctors at Corpus Christi, Texas, and they reviewed her medical record from Bethesda, they refused to believe that she had ever had thyroid nodules.

Aside from Dr. Stambul's and his own observations relative to the protective, life-extending power of the ovaries, Dr. Myers cites the dog experiments of Perkin and Brown of Lahey Clinic, Boston. After the thyroid gland of a male dog has been surgically removed, his protein-bound iodine plummets to one-tenth its normal level. After the same operation, a female dog's protein-bound iodine remains the same until the ovary is removed. Then it drops to the same level as that of the male.

Over and above being protected from cardiovascular problems by ovarian secretions, women are also protected against cystic fibrosis as well as cancer of the breast and ovaries. Dr. Myers states that iodine, tyrosine, vitamins, amino acids and trace minerals will guard a woman against numerous ailments, and that she should not give up her ovaries in panic at any point in her life, unless they have been proved to be cancerous. Then it is foolish to resist.

Many abnormal physical conditions result from inadequate diet, a good reason to examine our nutritional regimes for deficiencies and to be aware of the available array of helpful dietary supplements, new and old. One particular food supplement, evening primrose oil, fills a special niche and is a precursor to body substances which have many functions similar to those of thyroid hormones. This is the subject of the next chapter.

16

EVENING PRIMROSE OIL:
WONDER-WORKER

The more I read, the more excited I grew.

Twenty-two published reports covering clinical and double-blind studies of evening primrose oil had convinced me that this is the most remarkable all-purpose food supplement to burst onto the horizon in a generation.

And the more I read, the more I realized that evening primrose oil and thyroid hormone prevent and relieve an almost identical list of disorders: arthritis, cardiovascular ailments, premenstrual syndrome, skin problems such as acne, eczema and icthyosis, infection and inflammation, diabetic complications and certain other degenerative diseases which encourage faster aging.

Why do evening primrose oil and thyroid hormone seem to work effectively on many of the same disorders? Research needs to be done to offer a conclusive answer, although certain facts already seem clear. Prostaglandins (PGs), whose precursors are contained in the essential fatty acids (EFAs) in evening primrose oil, are present in infinitesimal amounts in every human cell and, though short-lived, exert a strong influence on every bodily function. Thyroid hormone, too, is carried through the bloodstream to every cell, where it governs life processes.

PGs, like thyroid hormone, are involved in blood circulation, in metabolism, in growth and reproduction and in proper function of the immune system. Individuals deficient in PGs catch every communicable disease. So do hypothyroids.

Aside from comparisons with thyroid hormone, evening primrose oil has an incredibly promising life of its own. It is important—even fundamental—for us to know exactly what it is and what it can do for us.

Evening primrose oil, which sounds like a beauty product that might be found in a woman's boudoir, is actually something that should be on her vitamin shelf as well as that of everyone in the household. It contains an essential fatty acid, a vitamin-like compound that can't be made in the human body. (That is what "essential" means in this context.) The World Health Organization suggests that adults should take in at least 3 percent of their total calories as EFAs; the figure is 5 percent for children and lactating women.

EFAs perform many functions; their chief roles are as integral parts of every membrane in the body and as the precursors of prostaglandins, key short-term regulators which help control all bodily organs.

Unless enough EFAs are supplied, physical abnormalities develop. These include defects in heart function and in circulation; subnormal complexion with acne and eczema; poor immune function; failure of wounds to heal; reproductive shortcomings or failure, particularly in men; inflammatory ailments and arthritis; infiltration of fat and fibrosis of the liver; failure of the brain to develop normally; imbalance of body water; and atrophy of exocrine (ducted) glands.

Can't we get enough EFAs from the usual sources of polyunsaturates? Not always. Not all polyunsaturates are biologically active. Vegetable oils are rich in linoleic acid, an essential raw material for prostaglandins, but coconut, olive and palm oil are not. Vegetable oils processed for cooking fats and margarines often lose their EFA activity and can even become anti-EFA factors. Human milk has a high content of linoleic acid; other foods have negligible amounts.

On its way to becoming PGs, linoleic acid must go through conversion to gamma-linoleic acid (GLA), then to dihomo-gamma-linoleic acid (DGLA).

Only breast-feeding infants can get GLA, DGLA and certain PGs directly; the rest of us must obtain them through the metabolism of ingested linoleic acid. Females are far better at converting this acid into GLA than males, so the latter require a larger intake.

A biochemical obstacle course blocks persons following a typical western lifestyle from forming GLA from linoleic acid: a diet heavy in saturated fats and cholesterol, processed vegetable oil and alcohol.[1] These impediments grow more daunting when added to the aging process and slower metabolism, virus infections, degenerative diseases, radiation and zinc deficiency.

Only nursing infants were privileged to get prostaglandin precursors and some PGs directly until recent scientific experiments revealed the remarkable biochemical values of evening primrose oil, which contains 8 to 9 percent GLA and more than 70 percent of cis-linoleic acid, the EFA-active form.[2]

Where has evening primrose oil been all our lives? It has been around for centuries, but was not fully appreciated until recently. For hundreds of years, the American Indians pressed the oil from seeds of the evening primrose, a lovely yellow eastern seaboard wildflower that blooms and dies in a single evening. They cured skin problems and wounds by applying this oil, and took it orally for asthma. Early colonizers of America shipped evening primrose oil plants back to England, where the flower achieved such healing success that it was called the King's cure-all.

From 1965 to 1981, Agricultural Holdings Ltd., a British seed company, conducted an extensive botanical search and found more than 1,000 varieties of evening primrose, from which they developed plants with the richest yield of consistently high quality oil.

The critical role of evening primrose oil in promoting the formation of prostaglandins has excited the scientific community.

Now there is a ready source of PG precursor to help realize the unlimited possibilities of prostaglandins to keep us healthy.

The explosion of publications about prostaglandins has reached unimaginable proportions: hundreds of papers in some months— far more than most physicians can read and still carry on a medical practice.

Like evening primrose oil, prostaglandins are not new. They were known more than fifty years ago and given their peculiar name because they were first discovered in semen in the prostate gland. In the 1960s—long after it was too late to put PGs through a legal name change—it was found that they are synthesized in almost every body cell. A decade after that, scientists learned that aspirin kills pain by blocking the production of two forms of PG.

By providing precursors of PGs, evening primrose oil has been discovered to be clinically valuable in a wide range of medical problems, including arthritis, cardiovascular ailments, premenstrual syndrome, breast pain, obesity, hyperactivity, diabetes, brittle nails, hair loss, skin diseases and allergies.[3] It was shown to be effective in controlling adjuvant arthritis in rats and rheumatoid arthritis in some human patients.[4]

Evening primrose oil also appears to lower the risk of heart attacks in animals and human beings. Its high content of EFAs keeps blood platelets from sticking together and forming clots, and helps lower blood cholesterol and blood pressure.

Evening primrose oil has also earned high marks in a disorder that plagues many women, premenstrual syndrome (PMS). Its symptoms include fluid retention, swollen ankles, painful breasts, pelvic congestion, abdominal bloating and mood disorders such as depression, irritability, headaches, weeping and, in some cases, uncontrollable rage.

In two experiments in Great Britain, evening primrose oil showed promise in preventing symptoms of PMS. At one of the world's largest PMS clinics, St. Thomas Hospital in London, M. G. Brush, M.D., administered primrose oil to seventy women who had failed to get relief from one or two other attempted treatments. Taking two capsules three times daily, 67 percent of the women were completely relieved of PMS symptoms. Twenty-two percent gained partial relief. A surprising total of 89 percent of treatment-resistant women experienced partial to total relief.[5]

At the Universities of Wales and Dundee, 100 women took part in a placebo-controlled double-blind crossover study with evening primrose oil to treat breast pain. (Many of the subjects experienced worse pain premenstrually.) A majority of the women experienced significant pain relief.[6]

In an area of concern to both women and men, evening primrose oil showed ability to help obese subjects lose weight. Among individuals more than 10 percent above ideal weight who took this supplement, 50 percent lost weight without a change of diet. Subjects who were within 10 percent of ideal body weight showed no weight change on evening primrose oil. Those who lost weight claimed they noted a reduced appetite without any effort on their part.[7]

Evening primrose oil has proved somewhat helpful in cases of alcohol addiction and much more so in lessening the harmful effects of alcohol. GLA, DGLA and PGE1, a critical prostaglandin, are depleted in alcoholics. Conversion of linoleic acid to GLA is blocked by alcohol, causing a functional lack of EFA, even though intake of linoleic acid seems to be sufficient. DGLA is rapidly used up, and the process of replenishment from linoleic acid is shut down.[8] After appreciable drinking, levels of the prostaglandin PGE1 drop down and bring on depression. In turn, depression predisposes the person to further drinking and to alcoholism—especially women, according to a scientific report. Evening primrose oil can help relieve the depression and discourage additional drinking. In one experiment, it prevented severe post-alcohol depression, tachyarrythmias (too-rapid heart action) and hangovers.[9]

Aside from seriously depleting GLA, DGLA and PGE1, alcoholism causes liver damage and kidney defects. Evening primrose oil has been shown to break the enzyme block caused by alcohol and to protect both liver and kidneys.

Rarely a disorder of adults, hyperactivity is a serious problem for children, their parents and teachers. Sometimes these "perpetual motion" children who are often classroom disturbers can be helped by the Feingold diet, which eliminates foods with additives and junk foods.

Food additives appear to offer weak resistance to the conversion of EFAs to PGs. One new theory holds that hyperactivity may be caused by subnormal intake of EFAs. (Thirst, common in this ailment, is a revealing symptom of EFA deficiency in animals.) Boys outnumber girls in hyperactivity by three to one. Inasmuch as boys have trouble converting EFA to PGs, they require about three times as much EFA as girls.

Preliminary studies of hyperactive children by clinicians in the United States, Canada, South Africa and the United Kingdom indicate that approximately two-thirds of the subjects improve after ingestion of evening primrose oil. A peculiarity noted in these experiments is that certain children responded better to the oil if it was rubbed into their skin. Researchers believe that this is true because some individuals have poor intestinal tract absorption. Dosages used were two to three capsules each morning and evening and, after six to eight weeks, one in the morning and one in the evening.[10]

In another disorder, diabetes, evening primrose oil helps in two ways, one immediate, the other long range. Experiments demonstrated that diabetic animals cannot readily convert linoleic acid to GLA. Presumably, the same thing happens in human beings. EFA supplementation often raises levels of linoleic acid, GLA, DGLA and certain prostaglandins in diabetics.

An EFA-rich regime also helps control long-term complications of diabetes. A five-year study of 102 diabetics at Erasmus University in Rotterdam used matched groups of patients, one on a normal diet, the other on a linoleic acid-enriched diet (13 percent of the calories). At the study's end, 62 percent of males and 55 percent of females on the normal diet developed retinopathy (deterioration of arteries in the retina that often impairs sight). Only 27 percent of males and 32 percent of females on the linoleic acid-enriched diet developed retinopathy.[11]

Essential fatty acids play a crucial role in the health and beauty of skin, hair and nails. When individuals are deficient in EFAs, or if EFAs cannot be translated into GLA (as is the case in zinc deficiency), skin lesions similar to those in eczema and ichthyosis (fish skin) develop, along with hair loss and brittle, cracking nails. Experiments have established that children with eczema have low levels of EFAs; it has also been shown that depriving children of EFAs leads to eczema.[12] Infants on mother's milk get preformed GLA, so the problem in forming this compound from linoleic acid is eliminated. The only other way to get preformed GLA is from evening primrose oil. Three capsules contain roughly the same amount of GLA as a day's supply of human milk. Marginal effectiveness of EFA in improving eczema may mean that the principal problem lies not in the amount of linoleic acid available but in the amount convertible to GLA.

A double-blind, placebo-controlled experiment at the University of Bristol in England showed that evening primrose oil brought about a modest but significant improvement in eczema of adults and children.[13] In a related condition, brittle and cracking nails, nails were dramatically improved by evening primrose oil; this was demonstrated in an experiment at Hairmyres Hospital in East Kilbride, Scotland. Dr. Allan Campbell, a prominent researcher, concludes that poor nails are a newly discovered symptom of EFA deficiency.[14]

With regard to a severe skin ailment, atopic eczema, a double-blind controlled cross-over study of different doses of evening primrose oil on ninety-nine patients revealed significant clinical improvements in high dosages with no side effects, according to a study reported in *Lancet.*[15]

Atopic eczema is one of numerous, often dissimilar diseases linked biochemically to one another—among them, allergies, asthma and hay fever—that are endured by some 40 million Americans. Several studies on atopic disorders show three prominent features: (1) They run in families; (2) atopics are deficient in certain essential blood ingredients, including elements for synthesizing prostaglandins; and (3) their immune system has deficiencies which reduce its effectiveness in dealing with threatening invaders.

Every minute of the day and night we are exposed to bacteria and viruses and to foreign substances in the air we breathe, the food we eat and the water we drink. Some of them are harmless; others are harmful. Our immune system must distinguish which is which and neutralize or destroy harmful invaders. T suppressor lymphocyte cells are the immune system's "field generals"; they issue orders as to which invaders to attack.

The best present scientific information holds that in atopic persons, the T suppressor cells are defective. The field generals are not competent to command. They are indiscriminate. Immune system soldiers under them blindly obey orders and attack harmless substances—foods such as eggs and milk proteins, as well as pollens, molds and animal dander—along with the real enemies.

This senseless warfare manifests itself in allergies, asthma, eczema and sometimes in headaches, when the brain is the battle area. Much current data indicates that prostaglandins control the T suppressor cells. A PG shortage in numbers and in specific types is believed to cause abnormal and harmful immune response. The protectors turn on the protected. It is no wonder that atopics are far more susceptible to infection and inflammation than normal individuals. The solution? Providing sufficient evening primrose oil.

Many authorities feel that a malfunctioning immune system, which makes a person illness-susceptible, also causes premature aging. Experiments show that animal aging is related to loss of ability to convert linoleic acid into GLA, which could account for cardiovascular and immune system abnormalities and degeneration. Studies are under way to determine if bypassing the body's need to translate linoleic acid into GLA by supplying evening primrose oil is a deterrent to aging. Time and research may soon provide the answer.

Slowing down the process of aging involves far more than just the immune system, conversion of linoleic acid into GLA and assuring the body sufficient thyroid hormones, as important as all these factors are. It involves a many-faceted approach, as the next chapter will illustrate.

17

LIVE LONGER, HEALTHIER AND YOUNGER

An alltime high in long-living was set by a fellow named Methuselah—969 years. He isn't mentioned in the *Guinness Book of World Records*, but you *can* find him in the Book of Genesis.

You may not expect to dethrone Methuselah, but wouldn't it be great to live several decades longer than average with great health and a sharp mind?

You *can*.

First, however, you should be armed with the latest solid information on this subject—psychological, social, physical and biochemical.

Staying young starts with thinking and acting young. A positive attitude helps because, sooner or later, signs of aging appear somewhere between the top of the head and the soles of the feet. It is essential not to let an unwelcome wrinkle, a gray hair, or a joint's worth of arthritis send negativism richocheting through your mind, causing you to give in to aging.

Accentuating the negative only accelerates the aging process, as it did in the forty-five-year-old father of a school acquaintance of mine back east. His frequent comment was, "I'm getting old fast."

Returning after a decade away, I was shocked at how cruelly the years had treated him. Yet there was grim justice in the physical response to his self-image. A comparatively youthful, vigorous middle-aged man had become bent, faltering and stiff-legged, his hands locked like claws with arthritis. Poor self-image and negative programming were surely not the only factors in his rapid deterioration, but they were powerful determinants.

Certain psychological and social factors contribute strongly to staying young, says Dr. G. Z. Pitskhelauri, a noted Russian gerontologist, based on in-depth studies in the Soviet Union's Republic of Georgia, reputedly the home of more hundred-year-olds (and older) than any other area in the world.[1]

Following are his major requirements for longevity, many of which can be applied in the United States: (1) close family ties—the branch should always remain a part of the family tree. If possible, several generations should live under a single roof; (2) a continuous daily work routine within the body's capabilities: (3) continued physical activity, not vegetative retirement; (4) independent pursuits within the close family structure; (5) periods of relaxation.

Dr. Pitskhelauri would take exception to Oliver Wendell Holmes's classic witticism that the best way to live long is to select your grandparents wisely. Environment is more important than heredity, at least so far as the Republic of Georgia is concerned, he maintains. In answer to the argument that many long-living Georgians also have long-living ancestors, he states that this is to be expected, because they are products of the same environment.

Dr. Pitskhelauri also says that a key to longevity is the typical Georgian diet, one that gives the back of the hand to the low-cholesterol diet: fatty meats, whole milk products, native sauces, herbs and other greens and moderate amounts of wine.

His final words of advice are to eat in moderation; avoid hard liquor and tobacco: be active, with a lively interest in family and the community; and, of crucial importance, follow regular life patterns (including work) and try to stay free of excess stress.

Another longevity program—this one in the United States—is based on a comprehensive survey by the California State Department of Public Health.[2] Several thousand individuals were interviewed initially and then nine years later. Persons who adhered to at least six of the following rules experienced better health and more years to enjoy it than those who complied with fewer than four:

1. Sleep seven to eight hours a night.
2. Always eat breakfast.
3. Snack infrequently.
4. Keep weight to between 5 percent under and 20 percent over desirable standard weight (for males) and less than 10 percent over desirable standard (for females).
5. Exercise frequently: do some physical work such as gardening; pursue sports (swimming, golf, calisthenics) and take long walks.
6. Always keep alcoholic consumption under five drinks on any one occasion.
7. Do not smoke.

Such guidelines offer a helpful pattern for longevity. However, certain bits of misinformation still mislead and discourage the young on their way to advanced years, as well as those who are already there. One of them is the moss-covered cliche, "You can't teach an old dog new tricks." Another is the belief that we inevitably begin losing irreplaceable brain cells at age twenty-six and with them essential mental capacity.

More than a generation ago, studies by Dr. Irving Lorge of Columbia University proved conclusively that old dogs not only learn new tricks but learn them well. A remarkable research project conducted by Dr. William A. Owens, Jr., while he was head of the psychology department at Iowa State University, exploded the "old dogs" cliche again. He happened upon a musty treasure in the attic of a college building—scores of 179 freshmen who, in 1919, had taken the Army Alpha test, one of the first comprehensive means of measuring mental ability. Aware that he could make a tremendous contribution to psychological knowledge, Dr. Owens managed to track down 127 of these then middle-aged individuals and administered the same test, comparing performances.

What impressed him most was that, after four years of college and three decades of experience, these individuals scored higher on general information and far higher on questions requiring judgment and logic. Unquestionably, the fifty-year-olds demonstrated superior thinking ability when compared with their younger selves.

In 1971 the Soviet Union issued a report to the United Nations, *The Right to Old Age*, based on tested physical and mental abilities of 21,000 elderly individuals. Its conclusion was, "The more brains and muscles are used, the less they age."

Many similar studies have been published in the past fifty years, and now scientists in laboratories are learning underlying reasons for previous findings.

One of the leaders in this alluring field of research is Professor Marian Diamond, a neuroanatomist at the University of California at Berkeley. Results of her twenty years of experiments with rats have given the world enlightenment and new hope. She says that if we seek stimulation and challenge all of our lives, we can delay and even defeat mental aging. She has also shattered the misconception that we necessarily lose thousands of brain cells daily, that there is nothing we can do to replace them and that therefore our mental capacity declines steadily and inevitably.[3]

To skeptics who might say, "All of this is helpful if you're a rat," Professor Diamond responds that brains are big clumps of nerve cells, and that nerve cells of rats and human beings have the same basic constituents. In the Gertrude Stein tradition, she says, "A nerve cell is a nerve cell is a nerve cell."

It is not true that the brain settles on a comfortable plateau of accomplishment in early life and declines after that. Professor Diamond learned that there can be brain growth even in rats who are in their 80s and 90s in human years. In one experiment, she moved rats who had lived boring lives in uninteresting cages with only a few companions into what she called "enriched quarters," with larger cages, a choice of toys, and sometimes twelve other rats for companionship. Toys were changed every day. She compared this group's progress with that of a control group, rats in standard dull cages with no toys and only two companions. Without stimulation or challenge, the control rats stayed in their rut, keeping to themselves, hardly moving, moping and acting as old as they were. It was just the opposite for the rats in the enriched environment. They socialized, played with their new toys and seemed to look forward to the next day's toys.

At the end of the experiment, when the rats were more than 120 years old in human terms, those in the enriched environment had actually increased their number of brain cells. Their cerebral cortex was 6 percent thicker than that of the unstimulated rats. Further, their brains showed 9 percent less lipofuscin (aging pigment).

Nerve cells were designed to receive stimuli. They will react positively to stimuli at any age, Professor Diamond says. Brains which meet challenges positively don't lose cells; they gain some. Professor Diamond sees a lesson for human beings in the rat studies. We can socialize, keep our minds stimulated and stay young or isolate ourselves, vegetate and age rapidly. The decision is up to us. It's a question of using or losing our brain power.

Other scientists worldwide are also uncovering secrets to keep us physically young for productive living. Most gerontologists agree that there's no point in extending life only to give ourselves an additional fifteen or twenty years to be ravaged by disease and degeneration.

Dr. Allan Goldstein, chairman of the biochemistry department of George Washington University Medical School, Washington, D.C., one of the foremost researchers in longevity, feels that scientists will soon discover how to use immune system energy, just as researchers decades ago learned how to release energy by splitting the atom. Effervescent with optimism, Dr. Goldstein feels that within a decade we will know how to live to 100 or beyond. It will be up to us to learn how to use this information.

How can immune system energy be utilized for our benefit? Before we answer, let us review what the immune system is and what it does. The immune system is an inner guard that protects us from threats to our existence, from anything that's foreign or abnormal, whether it is a transplanted organ or malaria germs, viruses or cancer cells.

A popular theory holds that when the immune system begins to decline, that is the beginning of the end. The decline appears to start in the thymus gland, a twin-lobed, gray-pink organ located at the top of the chest. Dr. Goldstein calls the thymus (thought to be useless until the early 1960s) the immune system's master gland. Unlike other glands whose peak productivity continues for many years, the thymus slows down when we are about fourteen years old.

Protective white blood cells called T-cells pass through the thymus gland to be modified and matured for action. These cells fight for our lives. Like soldiers, they have various missions— annihilating invaders, stimulating certain immune functions, shutting down others, enhancing the ability of antibodies (cells which provide immunity against disease) to recognize enemies. As a person ages, the immune system cells lose their power to protect against infection as well as their ability to distinguish between friends and enemies. Then they sometimes mistake their own body tissues for enemies, and attack. This is what happens in autoimmune disease.

When we reach the age of fifty, the immune system is operating on something like 15 percent of full efficiency. A weakened immune system loses its ability to monitor and kill abnormal cells; this is a cause for the growing threat of cancer as we grow older, according to some authorities.

As the thymus gland weakens, it is important that we supplement this organ as we do the lazy or weak thyroid gland. The main thrust of thymus research is therefore the synthesizing of a family of hormones named thymosins. The co-discoverer of thymosin, Dr. Allan Goldstein, says scientific evidence indicates that the immune system probably can be rejuvenated by thymosin. In experiments at the National Institutes of Health, these hormones proved effective in blocking, delaying and even curing certain cancers which seem age-related—those of kidney, lung and prostate.

A controlled study of fifty-five patients afflicted with inoperable oat cell lung cancer brought rewarding results. Thymosin supplementation doubled survival time. Twenty-one subjects received extremely high doses of this hormone and were cleared of cancer. Two years later they are still free of it.

Another authority on thymosin, Dr. William Regelson, professor of medicine and microbiology at the Medical College of Virginia, has had some encouragement in experiments with these hormones against rheumatoid arthritis and multiple sclerosis. He says that this approach is a fundamental one, aimed at the heart of the problem, not at the edges.

Thus far, the side effects of thymosin supplementation seem negligible. The body appears to use what is required from what is injected and excretes the rest.

Not all the world's best gerontologists agree by any means that the declining immune system is the sole cause of aging, important though it is. Some maintain that the individual cells gradually lose their ability to repair DNA, the complex chemical of heredity. Still another group feels that a buildup of free radicals accelerates aging. Free radicals are atoms with an unpaired or odd electron, or clusters of such atoms. They originate from chemicals in food, water and air, from radiation and from oxidation, which goes on ceaselessly in the cells. Highly charged with energy and as unpredictable as a violent person, they run amuck and attack, damage or destroy healthy cells.

Protection of body cells, in which an estimated thousand chemical processes go on, is accomplished by antioxidants, including vitamin C, a water-soluble nutrient; vitamins A and E, oil-soluble vitamins; selenium, a trace mineral which cooperates with vitamin E, and iodine.

The late Dr. Benjamin Frank believed that supplementary nucleic acids—DNA and RNA—protect cell integrity, too, and even reverse aging. The best sources of nucleic acids, which he advised taking with plenty of fluids, are brewer's yeast, sardines and leafy green vegetables. Nucleic acids supposedly minimize production of free radicals within cells.

Various authorities feel that high-quality nutrition, regular exercise and care of the heart and arteries contribute to longer life.

Dr. Linus Pauling favors taking in 8 to 10 grams of vitamin C daily, a practice which he believes may extend lifespan by twenty-four years.

Dr. Roy L. Walford of the University of California at Los Angeles advocates a severe restriction of food as one of the best ways to prolong life, particularly starting in the early years. His experiments with mice demonstrate the validity of his thesis.[4] While the Walford system appears to work, it is doubtful whether most individuals could endure his Spartan limitations without divine intervention. Furthermore, the pleasure of eating (not overeating) is part of our enjoyment of life.

Aside from deficiencies in critically needed vitamins, minerals, nucleic acids, and sometimes proteins, the greatest problem in nutrition for longer life is overeating and its natural consequence, obesity. As fat accumulates in all the old familiar places, chances of becoming a victim of brain disease, cancer, diabetes, gallbladder trouble, heart disease and liver ailments soar, says Dr. Grant Gwinup, professor of medicine at the University of California, Irvine.

"Stay active physically if you want to live long," insist advocates of daily exercise. Dr. Lawrence Morehouse, professor of exercise physiology at UCLA, states in his book *Total Fitness in 30 Minutes a Week* that 80 percent of the adult American population doesn't exercise properly or sufficiently to stop physical decay.

Although many authorities find that we benefit most from a lifetime of physical exercise, Dr. Herbert deVries, exercise physiologist at the University of Southern California Gerontology Center, insists that older people can also profit from exercise even if they start late in life. Men between ages of fifty-two and eighty-eight at Leisure World, a retirement colony at Laguna Hills, California, were put through carefully monitored exercise routines by Dr. deVries and showed surprising improvement: 35 percent greater breathing capacity and 30 percent increased ability of the blood to transport oxygen to tissues. They also realized greater ability to relax and to release pent-up feelings of frustration, aggression and hostility.

All too often, individuals who are indifferent to the needs of their body for exercise, rest and proper diet receive painful reminders in the form of degenerative diseases, including arthritis, one of the most exquisite tortures ever to twist and gnarl the human frame and appendages.

As early as the late nineteenth century, researchers found

thyroid supplements effective in managing arthritis in hypo-thyroids. They came to this knowledge by accident. In subnormal thyroid function, when the thyroid gland became enlarged and choked off the windpipe and breathing and doctors surgically removed the entire gland, they discovered that arthritis usually became worse. This valuable information was buried under the landslide of new scientific information. A Harvard University study showed that two-thirds of 312 patients with arthritis were hypothyroid. Dr. Loring P. Swaim, who was in charge of the project, suggested that arthritis develops in persons with low metabolism.[5]

Dr. Broda Barnes, following Dr. Swaim's lead, made a similar discovery in his study of 300 arthritics, and published his findings in a prestigious medical journal.[6]

"There is a characteristic pattern marking the patient with crippling arthritis," he once told me. "First, it is poor circulation, then repeated infections throughout the years and other symptoms that come from low thyroid function. In the late stage of this disease, thyroid therapy alone may not be entirely effective against arthritis, even though other characteristic symptoms of hypothyroidism may respond satisfactorily," he says.

Stubborn cases have responded with Dr. Barnes's daily administration of as little as 5 mg of prednisone, the least harmful of the corticosteroids. Aware of the dangers of corticosteroids, I approached this treatment carefully. However, I have had excellent results with it, too.

One convincing fact arises from various research projects: the best time to treat arthritis by thyroid therapy is before you have it or in its earliest stages.

Hypothyroidism is not the cause of all illness. In diagnosis, however, it should be considered as a possible basic cause until ruled out by accurate testing, a check of symptoms and a complete medical history.

Efficiency of your thyroid gland is not something to take for granted. Everyone's status can change, as we pointed out when discussing the thyroid's many subtle suppressants mentioned throughout this book, particularly in Chapter 3, Care and Feeding of the Thyroid.

With enough thyroid hormone circulating in your five quarts

of blood, you can fend off life-shortening infections, allergies and a negative outlook. You can stall or even stop debilitating degenerative diseases such as cardiovascular ailments.

Your heart will beat vigorously and regularly and pump a rich volume of blood through resilient, clean and smooth arteries to nearby and distant destinations, efficiently delivering food and oxygen to every cell and carrying off wastes.

All the information in this chapter and in previous ones will prove valuable in assuring that you live longer, healthier and younger. It would be well to remember, however, that even a normal thyroid gland slows down with the passing years, although at a much lesser rate than the thymus. Then, perhaps, it will need a little help from its friend: you!

Best of luck!

18

FOR DOCTORS ONLY

Aside from references cited, information in this chapter is based on standard, recognized books: *The Thyroid*, edited by Sidney C. Werner and Sidney H. Ingbar, Harper & Row, New York, 1971: *Vitamins in Endocrine Metabolism* by Isobel Jennings, Charles C. Thomas, Springfield, Illinois, 1970, and *Victory Over Diabetes* by William H. Philpott, Keats Publishing, Inc., New Canaan, Connecticut, 1983.

The unsuspected cause of many chronic problems whose causes baffle all of us in the field of clinical medicine can be readily diagnosed by means of the Barnes Basal Temperature Test.

I am referring to hypothyroidism, which affects every major organ and profoundly influences the efficiency of metabolism of every cell. Its symptoms are numerous and protean.

Suffice it to say that there is no clear-cut hypothyroid syndrome. The symptoms of hypothyroidism can mimic many of the physiologic disturbances we see on a day-to-day basis. To ignore the thyroid connection, however, is merely to treat our patients symptomatically and not to treat the underlying causative factors of their illness.

Simple examples of this are patients with recurrent infections who are chronically treated with antibiotics. These patients are frequently hypothyroid. As noted later in this chapter, this is in part due to the thyroid hormone's control of certain immune functions. I can cite many other examples but these are included in the section on thyroid physiology.

The most accurate way to diagnose hypothyroidism is by means of the Barnes Basal Temperature Test. More than a hundred years of research has established a definite relationship between subnormal temperature, no matter how slight, and hypothyroidism. Broda O. Barnes, M.D., Ph.D., refined the test. A clinical researcher in hypothyroidism for half a century, Dr. Barnes has published more than a hundred papers on his investigations in the most reputable medical journals. He has had a strong influence on my career as a physician.

Initially, I approached his work with more than a tincture of skepticism, despite the fact that full details of how he evolved the test and proved its reliability had been published in the respected *Journal of the American Medical Association*.[1]

Over several years, Dr. Barnes had correlated the basal temperature of more than 2,000 individuals with metabolic rate (BMR) tests which he had performed himself to minimize the possibility of skewing results, and with thyroid blood chemistry results. Through the years, he found a much higher correlation of negative BMR results and clinical hypothyroidism with basal metabolic temperature than with results of any other test. In addition, Dr. Barnes learned that many of these clinically hypothyroid patients actually had euthyroid blood tests.

Even the additional fact that the basal temperature test had appeared in the *Physician's Desk Reference* for years failed to satisfy my reservations about its validity. However, in the interest of fairness, I kept an open mind toward the test, which is carried out as follows: Shake down a thermometer before going to bed at night and leave it on the bedside table. Immediately upon awakening in the morning, insert the thermometer snugly in your armpit for ten minutes as you lie quietly in bed. In normal thyroid function, the temperature range reads 97.8 to 98.2 degrees. A lower temperature indicates probable hypothyroidism. The test should be done on two consecutive days. Women obtain the most accurate readings if not menstruating or on the second and third day of menstruation.

In 1978, shortly after a long-distance telephone interview with Dr. Barnes on the medical talk show I then hosted on a San Francisco radio station, I tried the test on myself, discovered a low basal temperature and each day took a small amount of natural desiccated thyroid. (Dr. Barnes and his more than one hundred followers use the natural form, as I do, on the premise that nature should know better than man, with all his synthetic chemicals, what is best for the body.) My energy level increased. My ability to concentrate improved dramatically and many minor, nagging symptoms disappeared.

Next, I began using the basal temperature test on a number of problem patients who had failed to respond to the usual medications. When indicated, I gave them thyroid supplementation. Their quick, positive response dissipated the last vestiges of my skepticism.

I will frequently start a new patient on thyroid therapy even if the thyroid lab work is normal, and I believe there is scientific justification to use it. Thyroid medication given to carefully screened patients is, in my experience, almost always helpful. I start all my patients on the equivalent of ¼ to ½ grain of the Armour desiccated thyroid preparation, and increase their dosage in ¼-½ grain increments every seven to ten days until a level that achieves the desired clinical results is obtained.

The dosage I use most commonly in adults is 1 to 2 grains. I have never put a patient on more than 4 grains of thyroid hormone per day, as in most of these patients we achieved the desired result with the smaller 1 to 2 grain dosage.

During the time my patients are titrated with a thyroid preparation, I have them check their basal temperatures before each visit. I refrain from increasing their dosage if their basal temperature goes above 98.2 degrees, or if their resting heart beat is above 85 per minute, or if on history they relate episodes of either constant jitteriness or palpitations. Fortunately, these symptoms are encountered infrequently. Once my patients are titrated on a proper dosage of the thyroid hormone and they are symptomatically improved, I see them a minimum of once every two to three months for a year to make sure they are still doing well clinically. This also rules out a placebo response. Although in most instances the use of thyroid medication alone is sufficient to correct many of the symptoms I will discuss, the effects are greatly amplified by the judicious use of applied clinical nutrition.

The main complaint I encounter from physicians is that the basal temperature test is unscientific; they feel that hypothyroidism can be diagnosed only by the standard laboratory blood work. That is exactly what I once thought. Now the basal temperature test is invariably the starting point of my three-pronged diagnostic approach. I relate temperature to patient symptoms and, of course, to medical history.

Today, the vast majority of physicians rely heavily on results of blood tests for diagnosing thyroid function, perhaps too heavily. I make this statement because many of my patients—and those of Dr. Barnes—have been declared euthyroid by blood tests and proved to be conclusively hypothyroid according to the basal temperature test, symptoms and medical history.

A Mayo Clinic study by Drs. Joseph C. Scott, Jr., and Elizabeth Mussey determined that the diagnosis of thyroid function should be done carefully and judiciously to avoid errors.[2] A patient considered to be mildly hypothyroid by one doctor may be regarded as euthyroid by a second physician, if conclusions are based on just one interview or test.

"No single test procedure will define the status of the thyroid gland," they write. "Further, any combination of methods may lead to erroneous interpretation or to inconsistent results. The clinician must have the faculty of correlating the clinical appearance of the patient with laboratory findings."

The subtle development of hypothyroidism, too, makes diagnosis difficult; this is graphically reported in an article by Drs. Mark Gold, H. Rowland Pearsall and A. Carter Pottash in *Diagnosis*.[3] Dr. Gold and his associates studied 250 consecutive inpatients admitted to a psychiatric hospital for evaluation and discovered that an often undetected cause of depression is hypothyroidism, whose symptoms overlap those of depression.

They state that thyroid hypofunction first appears in subclinical form (grade three) manifested by decreased energy and depressed mood. Next, the condition deteriorates to mild hypothyroidism (grade two) whose symptoms are fatigue, dry skin and constipation. Blood levels of thyroid hormone are usually still normal, however. Then comes overt hypothyroidism (grade one) which presents the classical signs: a measurable decrease in circulating thyroid hormone, extreme weakness, dry skin, coarsening of hair, constipation, lethargy, memory impairment, a sensation of cold, slowed speech, and weight gain.

"It is not correct to say that hypothyroidism is present or absent, rather that there are grades of thyroid function," write the doctors. They conclude that one of every ten patients with initial complaints of depressed mood or decreased energy may have subclinical hypothyroidism.

"In our experience, thyroid hormone replacement is more effective therapy for such patients than anti-depressant drugs," they state.

These physicians stress the need for careful evaluation of depressed patients who have not responded to conventional treatment or those with a family history of thyroid disease to determine if they are suffering from either hyperthyroidism or hypothyroidism.

Hypothyroidism is often such an extremely subtle disease that physicians misinterpret its symptoms, states Gerald S. Levey, M.D., an endocrinologist and chief of medicine at the University of Pittsburgh School of Medicine, in an article "Hypothyroidism: A Treacherous Masquerader" in *Acute Care Medicine* (May, 1984).

The correct diagnosis is frequently missed, because a broad range of symptoms is generally not associated with hypothyroidism, he says: musculoskeletal disorders such as severe muscle cramps, particularly at night; long-standing low back pain; hematologic disturbances (one-third to one-half of hypothyroids show some loss of blood cell mass, resulting in anemia); coagulability ailments: easy bruising, minor bleeding and menorrhagia; rheumatologic conditions: stiffness, arthralgias and paresthesias in hands and feet with accent on stiffness, rather than pain; myalgic complaints and synovial effusions, mainly in the knees; hyperuricemia; and a decrease in heart muscle contractility.

These conditions can be improved or reversed with thyroid hormone replacement, he says. Relative to routine screening for thyroid function, Dr. Levey states that this would not be cost effective, inasmuch as numerous factors, among them drugs and systemic states, affect such tests.

In my opinion, it is prudent for medical clinicians to be suspicious of any patient with a chronically low basal temperature and treat him or her for underactive thyroid before using toxic drugs and irreversible surgical procedures.

The importance of thyroid function to good health should not be underestimated. The thyroid gland is the largest endocrine gland in the human body. It weighs less than an ounce, secretes less than a teaspoon of hormone substance a year and controls the metabolic activity of all of our cells. As Dr. Barnes says, "Cellular health depends on three factors, a steady supply of nutrients, oxygen and thyroid hormones." The thyroid hormones stimulate oxidative metabolism, thereby increasing the oxygen consumption of every cell.

Thyroid hormone also stimulates protein synthesis, that is, the buildup of protein from amino acids. Protein is necessary for replacing worn-out cells and for the manufacture of enzymes, which moderate the speed at which biochemical reactions take place within the cells. Thyroid hormone potentiates the effect of other body hormones such as adrenaline, is necessary for the secretion of the sex-activating hormones such as the gonadotrophins of the pituitary gland and is, in large part, responsible for controlling the rate of absorption of nutrients in the gastrointestinal tract.

In hypothyroidism, blood cholesterol and triglycerides are higher than average, a condition often predictive of cardiovascular disorders. Thyroid supplementation causes them to decrease.

Thyroid hormone is partly responsible for production of a compound known as retinine, essential for visual acuity at night. It is also necessary for the synthesis or activation of specific enzymatic proteins within cells and for the translation and transcription of nucleic acids. The major sites of thyroid hormone activity are the cell membranes, mitochondria, ribosomes and neuclei.

Thyroid hormone stimulates both the sodium pump and the

glycolytic pathways, leading to oxidative phosphorylation in tissues such as the liver, kidneys and muscles.

Hypothyroids characteristically have thick and puffy skin, due to an accumulation of a mucin-like substance called hyalouronic acid, which binds water. The most frequent complaint of such patients is that they accumulate fluid. Powerful diuretics rid the body of this substance, but it returns as soon as the water pills are discontinued. Low thyroid individuals are usually the patients who can't lose weight unless they subject their bodies to the rigors of spas, exercise and a very low calorie diet.

The swollen features of hypothyroids are characteristically non-pitting fluid accumulations around the eyes, hands, ankles and feet. The skin is usually pale and cool, as a result of generalized blood vessel constriction. Low thyroid patients often complain of an inability to sweat even in great heat, and of being cold all the time. Their skin is often dry and coarse, because of decreased secretion of the sebaceous glands. As a result of diminished blood supply and decreased skin metabolism, their wounds heal slowly. This is particularly true in diabetics, many of whom tend to be hypothyroid.

Low-thyroid patients will frequently have severe hair loss. In the differential diagnosis of alopecia, hypothyroidism should always be a prime suspect. Nails grow slowly, tend to be weak and brittle and are usually striated both longitudinally and transversely.

The hypothyroid patient's heart is characterized by a low stroke volume and decreased cardiac output. To compensate for this, the body increases blood vessel resistance in the skin, resulting in the coolness and pallor already described. There may also be a compensatory increase in blood pressure and this, coupled with an increased cholesterol and triglyceride level, often predisposes the patients to an increased incidence of coronary artery disease.

Hypothyroidism may also cause EKG and blood chemistry changes mimicking heart attacks and other cardiovascular disorders. The most common electrocardiographic changes are flattening or invasion of the T-wave, particularly in lead 2, along with generalized low P-wave, QRS and T-wave amplitude. Non-specific T-wave flattening and sinus bradycardia are frequently seen.

Cerebral blood flow and oxygen consumption may be decreased in hypothyroidism. Renal and glomerular blood flow is slightly decreased.

The digestive changes in the low-thyroid patient are quite common and reflect the general sluggishness of every tissue, cell and organ. The hypothyroid's common problems are the loss of appetite with either no weight loss or an actual weight increase and decreased peristaltic activity of all gastrointestinal cells, often resulting in chronic constipation.

Gaseous distention is another frequent complaint. Should this be accompanied by colicky pain, indigestion and vomiting, it may be mistaken for a mechanical ileus or other related GI problems, and result in unnecessary surgery.

In certain cases, hypothyroidism may also contribute to an inability of the stomach to secrete enough acid for proper digestion, causing a general inability to resorb and utilize the essential nutrients calcium and vitamin B12. It has been estimated that true pernicious anemia occurs in 12 percent of the hypothyroid population.

Serum chemistry determinations of SGOT, LDH and CPK are frequently increased in hypothyroidism. These blood chemistries will generally return to normal in two to four weeks after thyroid hormone therapy is begun. They are thought to represent changes in enzyme metabolism and not hepatic or cardiovascular damage. Serum amylase levels may likewise be increased. This is often accompanied by a decrease in gallbladder motility. All too frequently gallbladder disease is diagnosed in these cases, and may again result in unnecessary surgery.

The digestive change in hypothyroidism may, in many cases, leave an investigating clinician with a false sense that GI absorption is normal or even increased, due to the fact that decreased absorption is often offset by a decrease in the patient's intestinal motility.

Neurologically, the hypothyroid individual often suffers decreased circulation to the brain, which may contribute to a generalized slowing of all intellectual functions, including speech. These persons frequently lack initiative and may even be described as slow-witted. Memory frequently appears impaired, with a decrease in the powers of retention and desire to think, and, frequently, an increased level of irritability. Reasoning power, however, is generally good. Questions may be answered slowly but with enthusiasm. Sleepiness is another common symptom.

Behavior in the hypothyroid patient may run the gamut from hyperactivity to lethargy, depending on how he or she responds to profound mental fatigue. Hypothyroidism should always be considered in the differential diagnosis of children who are hyperactive. Low-thyroid patients are often classified psychiatrically as paranoid personalities or depressive types. Thyroid hormone therapy has been studied intensively in depressed patients.

Hypothyroid individuals show a characteristic electroencephalogram: abnormally flat, low voltage or lacking alpha waves. They may therefore be diagnosed as suffering from a primary brain dysfunction or neurological disorder. Such EEG changes will generally revert to normal once the patients are treated with thyroid hormone. In severe cases of hypothyroidism, patients may be predisposed to epileptic seizure. Hypothyroidism should always be included in any differential diagnosis of epilepsy.

Many low-thyroid patients complain of night blindness. This condition is generally caused by a deficiency of the vitamin A metabolized retinine A, which requires thyroid hormone for its generation, and is generally reversible following the administration of vitamin A and thyroid hormone.

Slurred speech and hoarseness are likewise found occasionally in hypothyroidism, due to a buildup of mucopolysaccharides in the tongue and the larynx.

Vertigo, sensory neural hearing loss and Ménière's disease may also accompany hypothyroidism. Dry ears often occur because of decreased activity of the cerumen glands. Sore throats, dysphagia, nasal congestion and headaches are likewise frequent.

Women are particularly vulnerable to undetected hypothyroidism. Complaints of diminished libido and menstrual irregularity such as menorrhagia and metrorrhagia are common, as are menstrual cramping and amenorrhea. As a result, these women may be subjected to unnecessary D & Cs as well as hysterectomies.

Hypothyroidism in the prepubertal girl may be associated with delayed growth or delay of menarche, and, if prolonged, may give rise to premature vaginal bleeding and premature breast development.

Diagnosis of hypothyroidism during pregnancy is essential, inasmuch as animal studies and clinical investigations strongly indicate that thyroid hormone is essential to normal fetal brain development. It is likewise essential to rule out hypothyroidism in patients with either chronic undiagnosed infertility or multiple miscarriages, as first-trimester fetal loss in hypothyroidism is common, approaching 50 percent or more in certain studies.

Thyroid hormone deficiency in the prepubertal male may result in delayed gonadic development, delayed sexual maturation, and, in the adult, a decrease in sperm count and sperm motility. Men with decreased sperm motility who have hypothyroidism diagnosed as the underlying causative factor should never be treated with human chorionic gonadotropin (CG) or testosterone unless hypothyroidism has been effectively ruled out and the symptoms persist despite a year or more of adequate hormone replacement. Premature use of androgen therapy in the preadolescent may mask or further delay the onset of normal puberty. The most common complaint of the hypothyroid adult male involving the reproductive system is a general diminution of sex drive and libido. Suspect hypothyroidism in anyone who complains of a diminished libido.

Carbohydrate metabolism in hypothyroidism is characterized by a decreased release of glycerol from adipose tissue, diminished glucose absorption and a decreased availability of amino acids and glycerol for gluconeogenesis. There is also frequently a characteristic flat glucose tolerance curve in these people because of their inability to absorb glucose from the GI tract.

In addition, a high serum amylase level is found in severely hypothyroid patients and is considered to reflect chronic pancreatitis. The mechanism is thought to be related to hypothermia, which is known to be a cause of pancreatitis. Thus, diabetes mellitus, which has long been attributed to an insulin imbalance, should, by definition, encompass a concept of generalized pancreatic insufficiency which may be due in no small part to chronic hypothyroidism and superimposed nutritional imbalances, leading to a breakdown of pancreas production of bicarbonate, secretion of proteolytic enzymes and insulin production.

The possible mechanism of diabetes and the chronic metabolic disturbances of pancreatic insufficiency caused by an unsuspected hypothyroid condition have been elucidated by William Philpott, M.D., in his book *Victory Over Diabetes*, in the following terms: Hypothyroidism (1) ——➤gives rise to pancreatitis ——➤

gives rise to pancreatic insufficiency; which results in insufficiency of proteolytic enzymes ——→gives rise to amino acid deficiencies ——→contributing to greater deficiency of proteolytic enzymes which are manufactured from amino acids; (2) decreases the quality and quantity of insulin which is, in fact, built from amino acids; (3) decreases lipase activty ——→gives rise to increased fatty acids in the blood ——→increased arteriosclerosis and heart disease; (4) increases absorption through the gut of poorly digested protein particles ——→yields kinin or inflammatory reactions in body tissues and organs, giving possible rise to atherosclerosis and/or severe mental changes, if the reactions take place in the brain, and also an increased absorption of circulating blood lipids into the arterial intima, possibly resulting in arteriosclerotic plaque; (5) decreases the production of pancreatic bicarbonate which is necessary for the alkaline medium of the small intestine ——→giving rise to metabolic acidosis after meals, since the pancreatic bicarbonate or HCO_3 has not neutralized the stomach acid as it empties into the duodenum ——→ giving rise to further effective reduction of any pancreatic proteolytic enzymes, as they require an alkaline medium in the small intestine to function best.

More than 80 percent of insulin-dependent diabetics had abnormal output of proteolytic enzymes, and most diabetics of more than five years' duration had an abnormal bicarbonate secretory response.

Drug metabolism is frequently changed in hypothyroidism. Such drugs as Digoxin are increased in the plasma, due to an increase in the half-life caused by a decreased glomerular filtration, as well as a decrease in peripheral metabolism. Drug therapy in hypothyroid patients should be undertaken with particular judiciousness. In fact, caution should be exercised with any patient, because so much hidden hypothyroidism exists.

Decreased thyroid function retards growth and delays maturation of the skeletal system, and this can be largely prevented or corrected by administration of the desiccated thyroid preparation.

Hypothyroid patients may complain of vague muscular and articular pains as well as coldness and stiffness of the extremities that resembles fibrositis and rheumatoid arthritis. Clinically, they may present with a laxity of the ligament capsules and tendons, causing joint instability, aching on motion, joint stiffness and pain. Symptoms are often worse in the morning or after immobilization and are exacerbated by cold and dampness. Infrequently, the hypothyroid patient presenting with musculoskeletal problems is found to have the characteristic articular deterioration of the person who has rheumatoid arthritis.

One study of hypothyroid patients in regard to the musculoskeletal system shows that nine of eleven test subjects had generalized osteoporosis. Another study revealed that 10 percent of persons with low thyroid function had an increased incidence of carpal tunnel syndrome. There tends to be an increased uric acid level in hypothyroid patients with musculoskeletal problems and generally an increase in their sedimentation rate, so these lab studies, although abnormal, may be misleading.

Muscle condition in hypothyroids may differ appreciably, from normal strength and firm to weak and flabby. Transient pain, stiffness and cramps—frequent complaints—are often due to mineral imbalances caused by this ailment.

A high percentage of hypothyroid patients suffer from iron-deficiency anemia. The hypoplastic anemia of the low thyroid patient is brought about by decreased production of circulating blood cells as an adaptive response to decreased tissue oxygen needs. In other words, diminished tissue oxygen consumption gives rise to a decrease in tissue hypoxia, which is a normal trigger for erythropoetin, which, under normal circumstances, increases the number of circulating red blood cells. There is, therefore, a decrease in iron turnover.

This type of anemia strongly resembles an adaptive anemia and the protein-calorie malnutrition which is frequently superimposed on it, and may further cloud the clinical picture. In general, though, the hypoplastic anemia of hypothyroidism is mild, with hemoglobin levels above 9 grams per 100 mls. A hemoglobin below 9 should cause suspicion that the anemia of the hypothyroid patient is perhaps superimposed on another type of anemia.

Environmental factors play a large role in thyroid functioning. Sulfonamide drugs have a potent antithyroid effect, as do all antidiabetic drugs. These inhibit the formation of thyroid hormone by inhibiting iodine uptake. Adrenal corticosteroids, too, have a depressing effect on thyroid function. Again, corticosteroids, Prednisone and the like, should be used judiciously in the patient with known hypothyroidism or with a suspected hypothyroid condition.

Defining hypothyroidism as purely an endocrine dysfunction is narrow and myopic in that the primary problem may not be in the glandular secretions themselves, but rather due to impaired cell surface binding, so that the physiology of these cells is abnormal even with a normal range of thyroid hormone.

In addition, different tissue types often have different responses to the same level of thyroid hormone so that, due to biochemical individuality, a thyroid hormone level within normal limits may be adequate for the smooth physiological function of a person's skeletal muscle, but be inadequate for optimal cardiac physiology. Also, the symptoms of subclinical hypothyroidism such as chronic fatigue, depression, mild anemias, inability to lose weight and the like, may be easily mistaken for a host of other disorders and written off as a neurotic or psychosomatic complaint.

Thyroid hormone is secreted into the bloodstream predominantly bound to three proteins: thyroid binding protein, thyroid binding prealbumin and albumin. Only a minuscule percentage of the thyroid hormone is active at the peripheral tissues in a free form. It is therefore possible, because of biochemical individuality, for the body to have an adequate total output of thyroid hormone but to be hypothyroid, because more than the optimal amount of hormone for a particular individual is bound by protein and therefore inactive. It is also possible, because of the liver's role in the T4-to-T3 conversion, to have an over- or under-conversion of T4 as a result of liver function. Patients with conditions such as hepatitis or the nephrotic syndrome will often have an accompanying thyroid dysfunction. In short, there is a difference in the output of thyroid by the gland and the level of activity of that hormone.

It is probably true that the parameters of normal that we now use in the diagnosis of thyroid illness are not wide enough to pick up the vast amount of hypothyroid pathology that exists. Some researchers suggest that the lower unit of the total T4 range be around 65 to 70 mcg per liter rather than the present 50, because of what was found to be a five times greater prevalence of hypothyroidism at the level of 65 mcg. This same determination has been made with all other commonly measured parameters of thyroid hormone with the same results.

It is apparent, therefore that the blood test criterion for thyroid disease should never be the be-all or end-all in the diagnosis of hypothyroidism, but rather just one parameter.

Elsewhere in this book, it was explained that the body's basal temperature is one of the most sensitive indicators of thyroid hypofunction. It is therefore clinically more accurate than blood tests in those patients whose symptoms are highly indicative of low thyroid but whose blood work says otherwise.

In accordance with research by Dr. Jeffrey Bland's group in Bellvue, Washington, there are certain other blood test criteria to corroborate the hypothyroid diagnosis with the Barnes Basal Temperature Test: (1) cholesterol in excess of 252; (2) a triglyceride level greater than 200; (3) a total CPK level above 30; (4) a BUN-to-creatinine ratio less than 12; (5) an LDH level greater than 40; (6) a cholesterol-to-HDL level greater than 5; and (7) an increased B-2 fraction in lipoprotein electrophoresis.

Pharmacologic doses of estrogen depress the secretion of thyroid hormone by suppressing TSH. This is very important in the population of women on oral contraceptive pills. Dr. Barnes's research indicates that many women who are taking birth control pills develop cardiovascular difficulties because of their underactive thyroid condition and not as a result of the side effects of the birth control medication itself.

The biologic reducing agents cystine and glutathione can markedly inhibit the thyroid gland's function. Cystine and glutathione are two of the major components of the glucose tolerance factor molecule which is necessary for carbohydrate metabolism.

There is some clinical evidence to show that massive doses of vitamin C can inhibit the thyroid by changing the ionization reactions in the thyroid gland proper. The B vitamin PABA, likewise, if taken in large doses, has an inhibitory effect on the thyroid gland.

The cyanide molecule is a potent inhibitor of the thyroid. Cigarette smoking can increase the body's concentration of certain cyanide-containing molecules. So cigarette smoking, in addition to all the other things we know about, can, in some cases, cause a fairly powerful inhibition of the thyroid gland.

AFTERWORD

There are always some people whose symptoms seem to indicate hypothyroidism but whose physical exam, clinical lab results and Barnes Basal Temperature Test are all within normal limits.

You may be one of them. Should you then consult your nearest psychiatrist? The answer is, "Possibly." We all have unfinished business psychologically. In certain instances, these problems may be converted into physical complaints. A purely psychological diagnosis is always one of exclusion. I will never tell a patient, "It's all in your mind," before attempting to rule out as many of the unsuspected causes of illness as I can, because—let's face it—a psychiatric diagnosis follows you around forever. Unfortunately, there are no recovered schizophrenics in the eyes of many employers. Once you've had a "nervous breakdown," you're always suspect by the narrow minds that pass uneducated judgment about everything.

The following are the main unsuspected causes of illness that I have encountered professionally. These should be checked into if the thyroid solution discussed in the book does not solve your own particular clinical problems.

1. Chronic auto-immune thyroiditis is a condition in which we probably produce antibodies to our own thyroid gland. Authorities currently estimate the incidence of thyroiditis to be about 69 per 100,000 population, which is a ten-fold increase since 1935. The overwhelming majority of cases of this disorder are women. The most common complaints of women with thyroiditis include: (1) profound fatigue which no amount of sleep seems to alleviate; (2) severe and unexplained depression, often coupled with emotional instability—anxiety and panic attacks— for which there is seemingly no external cause; (3) short term problems with memory and recent recall.

If you suffer from any or all of these specific symptoms, make sure your doctor orders two laboratory blood tests which will definitely diagnose this condition. These are (1) the anti-microsomal antibody test and (2) the anti-thyroglobulin antibody test, both of which should be performed by the Nichols Lab in southern California. A positive result on one or both of these tests is generally diagnostic of thyroiditis. In this instance, you had best see a specialist in endocrinology, who will follow your case and help stabilize your condition. (Note: I have recently seen two severely depressed young women who were close to checking themselves into a psychiatric unit in a local hospital until it turned out that they both had positive anti-thyroid antibody studies, diagnostic of thyroiditis. They are presently being treated primarily by an endocrinologist, inasmuch as the cause of their condition was physical and not psychological.)

You should be aware that a small but ever-increasing number of psychiatrists is becoming more concerned with the physical components of psychological complaints and will often order the tests I have mentioned. These individuals are known as orthomolecular psychiatrists. and they are represented by an organization known as the Orthomolecular Psychiatry Association. For more information about them, send a self-addressed, stamped, business-size envelope to Ortho-Psych, P.O. Box 1549, Lafayette, CA 94549-1549.

(2) Another major unsuspected cause of clinical problems is food and environmental allergies. These allergies, beyond any doubt, mimic most of the disorders discussed elsewhere in this book. If treatment of patients' hypothyroidism, coupled with an optimal nutritional program, is not getting the proper clinical results, I always test them for food and environmental allergies and sensitivities or refer them to a physician who specializes exclusively in this area, a clinical ecologist. You may get more information about clinical ecologists in your area by writing to me % Solved-Ecology, P.O. Box 1549, Lafayette, CA 94549-1549.

(3) Candida albicans is an insidious yeast infection which is growing in epidemic proportions. It affects mainly women in their childbearing years but can strike anyone—even infants. It assumes a wide variety of symptoms and can cause untold distress. Common major symptoms of chronic yeast infection include fatigue, poor memory, "spacy" feelings, depression, joint swelling or pain, constipation, diarrhea, bloating, impotence, endometriosis and premenstrual tension.

Candida victims can fight back by using a combination of diet, food supplements and drugs. You may obtain more information about yeast infections and how to deal with them by reading either *Candida Albicans* by Wunderlich and Kalita, one of Keats Publishing's Good Health Guides, or *The Yeast Connection* by William G. Crook, published by Professional Books, P.O. Box 3494, Jackson, Tenn. 38301.

(4) Adrenal exhaustion is a condition which may preclude substantive improvement of your symptoms. Your own nutritionally oriented physician may be able to help strengthen your adrenals by placing you on a small amount of hydrocortisone (5 mg four times a day, after meals and at bedtime). This regimen has been clinically tested for 25 years by William McKendree Jeffries, M.D., and I urge you to have your doctor read Professor Jeffries' book, *The Safe Uses of Cortisone*, published by Charles C. Thomas, which documents why and how to use cortisone to help restore you to peak health.

REFERENCES

Chapter 1

1. Herman H. Rubin, *Glands, Sex, and Personality* (New York: Wilfred Funk, Inc., 1952), 36.

2. Louis Berman, *The Glands Regulating Personality* (New York: The Macmillan Company, 1921), 55.

3. J. C. Scott, Jr., and Elizabeth Mussey, "Menstrual Patterns in Myxedema," *American Journal of Obstetrics and Gynecology* (1965): 90:161.

4. B. Stone, *American Medical News*: May 23, 1980.

5. E. R. Pinckney, "The Accuracy and Significance of Medical Testing," *Archives of Internal Medicine* (March, 1983): 143:3, 512.

6. A. S. Jackson, "Hypothyroidism," *Journal of the American Medical Association* (1957): 121–165.

7. Roger J. Williams, *Free and Unequal* (Austin, Tex.: University of Texas Press, 1953), 19.

8. J. C. Wren, "Thyroid Function and Coronary Atherosclerosis," *Journal of the American Geriatric Society* (1968): 16:696–704.

9. H. L. Newbold, *Dr. Newbold's Revolutionary New Discoveries About Weight Loss* (New York: Rawson Associates Publishers, Inc., 1977), 220–221.

Chapter 2

1. News Story, University of Mississippi Medical Center, Jackson, Miss., May, 1983.

2. Roger J. Williams, *Free and Unequal* (Austin, Tex.: University of Texas Press, 1953), 19.

3. Nathan Masor, *The New Psychiatry* (New York: Philosophical Library, 1959), 99–100.

4. *Ibid.*, 102, 103.

5. *Ibid.*, 105.

6. "Age and the Thyroid Gland," *Prevention* (August, 1971): 166.

Chapter 3

1. Isobel W. Jennings, *Vitamins in Endocrine Metabolism* (Springfield, Ill.: Charles C. Thomas, 1970), 41.

2. *Ibid.*

3. *Ibid.*, 45.

4. *Ibid.*, 65.

5. *Ibid.*

6. *Ibid.*

7. *Ibid.*, 75.

8. *Ibid.*, 80

9. *Ibid.*, 69.

10. *Ibid.*, 47.

11. *Ibid.*, 62.

13. *Ibid.*, 80.

14. *Ibid.*, 92.

15. *Ibid.*, 99.

16. *Ibid.*, 109.

Chapter 4

1. *Complete Book of Vitamins* (Emmaus, Pa.: Rodale Press, 1976), 507.

2. *Ibid.*, 507, 508.

3. *Encyclopedia of Common Diseases* (Emmaus, Pa.: Rodale Press, 1976), 44.

4. Noel K. Marshall, "A Chilling Effect," *Psychology Today* (February, 1982): 92.

5. *Ibid.*

6. Boris Sokoloff, *Middle Age is What You Make it* (Garden City, N.Y.: Garden City Publishing Company, 1942), 124.

7. E. Atkins, "Fever—New Perspectives on an Old Phenomenon," *New England Journal of Medicine* (April 21, 1983): 308:16, 958.

8. *Ibid.*

9. *Ibid.*, 958, 959.

10. *Ibid.*, 959.

11. Broda O. Barnes and Lawrence Galton, *Hypothyroidism: The Unsuspected Illness* (New York: Thomas Y. Crowell Company, 1976), 102.

Chapter 5

1. A. H. Curtis and John W. Huffman, *A Textbook of Gynecology* (Philadelphia and London: W. B. Saunders Company, 1950), 148.

2. E. S. Taylor, *Essentials of Gynecology* (Philadelphia: Lea & Febiger, 1969), 462.

3. *The Thyroid Gland* (Chicago: Armour Laboratories, 1945), 71.

4. P. Ylostalu et al., "Amenorrhea With Low Normal Thyroid Function and Thyroxine Treatment," *International Journal of Gynecological Obstetrics* (1980): 18:3, 176–80.

5. L. S. Matveewa, "Effect of Thyroliberin on the Prolactin Level in the Blood Serum of Primary Hypothyroid Patients,"- *Problems of Endokrinology* (1980): 26.5. 22–25.

6. P. Peczely et al., "Interrelationship Between Thyroid and Gonadal Function in Female Japanese Quail Kept Under Short and Long Photoperiods," *Journal of Endocrinology* (1980): 87 (1), 55–63.

7. B. K. Vonderhaar and A. E. Greco, "Lobulo-Alveolar Development of Mouse Mammary Glands Is Regulated by Thyroid Hormones," *Endocrinology* (February, 1979): 104 (2) 409–418.

8. Broda O. Barnes and Lawrence Galton, *Hypothyroidism: The Unsuspected Illness* (New York: Thomas Y. Crowell, 1976) 135.

9. Emil Novak, *Gynecology and Female Endocrinology* (Boston: Little, Brown and Company, 1941), 465.

10. Broda O. Barnes, "Making the Pill Safer with Thyroid." *Federation Proceedings* (March, 1970): 29:2.

11. Kaufman, David W. et al., "The Effects of Different Types of Intrauterine Devices on the Risk of Pelvic Inflammatory Disease," *JAMA* (Aug. 12, 1983): 250:6, 759–762.

Chapter 6

1. Webster-Barnes Foundation Conference on Thyroid (Dallas, June 6-7-8, 1980).

2. *Ibid.*

3. *Ibid.*

4. *Ibid.*

5. *Ibid.*

6. A. Aakvaag et al., "Hormonal Changes in Serum in Young Men During Prolonged Physical Stress," *European Journal of Applied Physiology* (October 20, 1978): 39:4, 283-91.

7. Sidney C. Werner and Sidney H. Ingbar, eds., *The Thyroid* (New York: Harper & Row, 1965), 765.

8. Peter A. Singer, "Effects of Hypothyroidism and Hyperthyroidism on Sexual Function," *Medical Aspects of Human Sexuality* (August, 1981): 15:8, 56R.

Chapter 7

1. Roy G. Hoskins, *The Biology of Schizophrenia* (New York: W. W. Norton & Company, Inc., 1946), 110.

2. Broda O. Barnes and Lawrence Galton, *Hypothyroidism: The Unsuspected Illness* (New York: Thomas Y. Crowell Company, 1976), 79.

3. Nathan Masor, *The New Psychiatry* (New York: Philosophical Library, Inc., 1959), 45.

4. Edward R. Pinckney and Cathey Pinckney, *The Fallacy of Freud and Psychoanalysis* (Englewood Cliffs, N.J.: Prentice-Hall, Inc., 1965), 101–102.

5. M. B. Whybrow et al., "Mental Changes Accompanying Thyroid Gland Dysfunction," *Archives of General Psychiatry* (1969): 20:48.

6. Barnes and Galton, *Hypothyroidism*, 82.

7. Masor, *Psychiatry*, 21.

8. Cathryn Elwood, *Feel Like a Million* (New York: Devin-Adair Co., 1956), 235.

9. J. M. Holmes, *British Medical Journal:* 5006: 1394–98.

10. Masor, *Psychiatry*, 20.

Chapter 8

1. Mark Gold, "Significant Number of Depressives May Have Hypothyroidism," *Family Practice News* (November, 1982): 1.

2. A. Coppen, P. C. Whybrow et al., "The Comparative Antidepressant Value of L-Tryptophan and Imipramine With and Without Attempted Potentiation by Liothyronine," *Archives of General Psychiatry* (1972): 26:234–241.

3. K. Jensen et al., "Depression," *Lancet* (November 8, 1975): 920.

4. P. L. Rabin and D. C. Evans, "Exophthalmus and Elevated Thyroxine Levels in Association with Lithium Therapy," *Journal of Clinical Psychiatry* (October, 1981): 398–400.

Chapter 9

1. Carlton Fredericks and Herman Goodman, *Low Blood Sugar and You* (New York: Constellation International), 18–23.

Chapter 10

1. *Encyclopedia of Common Diseases* (Emmaus, Pa.: Rodale Press, 1976), 461.

2. "Conference on Diabetes and Obesity," *The Sciences* (June, 1967): 7:1, 13, 14.

3. "Diabetes," United Press International release (November 21, 1981).

4. "Roles of Nutrition, Obesity, and Estrogen in Diabetes Mellitus: Human Leads to an Experimental Approach to Prevention," *Preventive Medicine* (1981): 10, 577–589.

5. William H. Philpott and Dwight K. Kalita, *Victory Over Diabetes* (New Canaan, Conn.: Keats Publishing, Inc., 1983), 56-65.

6. C. D. Eaton, "Co-Existence of Hypothyroidism with Diabetes Mellitus," *The Journal of the Michigan Medical Society* (1954): 53:1101.

Chapter 12

1. *Time* (March 26, 1984), 58–59.

2. *Modern Medicine* (March 1, 1984), 268.

3. L. V. Malysheva, "Tissue Respiration Rate in Certain Organs in Experimental Hypercholesteremia in Atherosclerosis," *Federation Proceedings* Translation Supplement (1964): 23:T562.

4. I. B. Friedland, "Investigations on the Influence of Thyroid Preparations on Experimental Hypercholesterolemia and Atherosclerosis," *Zeitung Ges. Exp. Med.* (1933): 87:683.

5. Broda O. Barnes and Charlotte W. Barnes, *Heart Attack Rareness in Thyroid-Treated Patients* (Springfield, Ill.: Charles C. Thomas Publisher, 1972), 75.

6. *Ibid.*, 76.

7. Edward R. Pinckney and Cathey Pinckney, *The Cholesterol Controversy* (Los Angeles: Sherbourne Press, 1973), 7–8.

8. *Los Angeles Times* (October 2, 1975): Section 1, page 2.

9. Richard Passwater, *Supernutrition for Healthy Hearts* (New York: Dial Press, 1976), 57.

10. M. K. Gersovitz, K. Motil, H. N. Munro, N. S. Scrimshaw, and V. R. Young, *American Journal of Clinical Nutrition* (1982): 35(1): 6–14.

11. Pinckney, E. and C., *Cholesterol*, 36.

12. *Journal of the American Medical Association* (June 8, 1964): 188:845.

13. Pinckney, E. and C., *Cholesterol*, 33.

14. *Ibid.*

Chapter 13

1. Broda O. Barnes and Charlotte W. Barnes, *Heart Attack Rareness in Thyroid-Treated Patients* (Springfield, Ill.: Charles C. Thomas, 1972), 25–27.

2. Frank Chappell, "Obesity Rather Than Diet Blamed in High Cholesterol," American Medical Association news story (October 25, 1976).

3. L. M. Hurxthal, "Blood Cholesterol and Thyroid Disease," *Archives Internal Medicine* (1934): 53:825.

4. Meyer Bodansky and Oscar Bodansky, *The Biochemistry of Disease* (New York: The Macmillan Company, 1940), 341.

5. J. D. Wilson et al., "Influence of Dietary Cholesterol in Cholesterol Metabolism," *Annals New York Academy of Science* (1968): 149:808–821.

6. Timothy G. Johnson and Stephen Goldfinger, *The Harvard Medical School Health Letter Book* (New York: Warner Books, 1981), 229–230.

7. William B. Kountz, *Thyroid Function and Its Possible Role in Vascular Degeneration* (Springfield, Ill.: Charles C. Thomas, 1951).

8. Mark Bricklin, *The Practical Encyclopedia of Natural Healing* (Emmaus, Pa.: Rodale Press, 1976), 196.

9. *The Complete Book of Vitamins* (Emmaus, Pa.: Rodale Press, 1977), 314–315.

10. *Ibid.*, 315–316.

11. *Ibid.*, 198.

12. Bricklin, *Practical Encyclopedia*, 310–311.

Chapter 14

1. *The Encyclopedia of Common Diseases* (Emmaus, Pa.: Rodale Press, 1976), 667–670.

2. *Ibid.*

Chapter 15

1. J. G. C. Spencer, "The Influence of the Thyroid in Malignant Disease," *British Journal of Cancer* (1954) 8:393.

2. *The Encyclopedia of Common Diseases* (Emmaus, Pa.: Rodale Press, 1976), 294–295.

3. H. Vorheer, "Thyroid Disease in Relation to Breast Cancer," *Klinical Wochenschr.* (December, 1978): 23-56, 1139–45.

4. D. P. Rose and T. E. Davis, "Plasma Triiodothyronine Concentration in Breast Cancer," *Cancer* (April, 1979): 43–4, 1434–8.

5. S. Shapiro et al., "Use of Thyroid Supplements in Relation to the Risk of Breast Cancer," *Journal of the American Medical Association* (October 10, 1980): 15–244, 1685–7.

6. J. C. Pita, Jr. et al., "Diminution of Large Pituitary Tumor After Replacement Therapy for Primary Hypothyroidism," *Neurology* (August 29, 1979): 29:8, 1169–72.

7. L. A. Guerrero and R. Carnovale, "Regression of Pituitary Tumor After Thyroid Replacement in Primary Hypothyroidism," *Southern Medical Journal* (April, 1983): 76:4, 529–31.

8. John A. Myers with Carl H. Schutte, *Metabolic Aspects of Health: Nutritional Elements in Health and Disease* (Kentfield, Cal.: Discovery Press, 1979).

Chapter 16

1. R. R. Brenner, "Metabolism of Endogenous Subtrates by Microsomes," *Drug Metabolism Review* (1977): 6:155–212, and D. F. Horrobin, "A

Biochemical Basis for Alcoholism-Induced Damage," *Medical Hypotheses* (1980): 6:929–42.

2. "Essential Fatty Acids (EFAs)—Measuring Deficiency," *Technical Information Bulletin #2:* Health from the Sun Products, Inc., New York, 1.

3. *Ibid.*, 2.

4. S. Kunkel, R. B. Zurier, "Treatment of Adjuvant Arthritis with Evening Primrose Oil," *Progress in Lipid Research*, in press.

5. M. G. Brush, "Efamol in Treatment of the Premenstrual Syndrome," Report for St. Thomas Hospital Medical School, London.

6. N. L. Pashby et al., "A Clinical Trial of Evening Primrose Oil (Efamol) in Mastalgia," presented at British Surgical Research Society, Cardiff (Wales) Meeting, July, 1981.

7. K. S. Vaddadi and D. F. Horrobin, "Weight Loss Produced by Evening Primrose Oil Administration in Normal and Schizophrenic Individuals," *IRCS Journal of Medical Science* (1979): 7:52.

8. D. F. Horrobin, "A Biochemical Basis for Alcoholism and Alcohol-Induced Damage," *Medical Hypothesis* (1980): 6:929–942, and Horrobin and M. S. Manku, "Possible Role of Prostaglandin E1 in the Affective Disorders and in Alcoholism," *British Medical Journal* (1980): 1:1363–6.

9. J. Rotrosen, D. Mandio, D. Segarich et al., "Ethanol and Prostaglandin E1: Biochemical and Behavioral Interaction," *Life Science* (1980): 26: 1867–76.

10. "Essential Fatty Acids and Hyperactivity," *Technical Information Bulletin #8:* Health from the Sun Products, Inc., New York, 1.

11. A. J. Houtsmuller et al., "Favourable Influence of Linoleic Acid on the Progression of Diabetes Micro- and Macroangiopathy," *Nutrition Metabolism* (1980): 24 (Supp. 1) 105–18.

12. A. E. Hansen, "Serum Lipid Changes and Therapeutic Effects of Various Oils in Infantile Eczema," *Proceedings of the Society of Experimental Biological Medicine* (1933): 31: 160–161, and A. E. Hansen and M. E. Haggard et al., "Essential Fatty Acids in Human Nutrition," *Journal of Nutrition* (1958): 565–76.

13. C. R. Lovell, J. L. Burton and D. F. Horrobin, "Treatment of Atopic Eczema with Evening Primrose Oil," *Lancet* (1981): 1:278.

14. A. C. Campbell, G. C. MacEwen, "Treatment of Brittle Nails and Dry Eyes," *British Journal of Dermatology*, in press.

15. *Lancet*, Vol. 1 (1981), 278.

Chapter 17

1. G. Z. Pitskhelauri, "The Long-Living of Soviet Georgia," *The Gerontologist* (February, 1982): 22:2, 117–118.

2. *Nutrition and the M.D.* (October, 1981): 7:10, 5.

3. "Keep Your Brain Young at Any Age," *Los Angeles Times* (April 26, 1983): Part 3, 1-4.

4. "Of Life Extension, Mice and Men," *Los Angeles Times* (June 21, 1982).

5. L. P. Swaim, "Chronic Arthritis," *Journal of the American Medical Association* (1929): 93:259.

6. Broda O. Barnes and Lawrence Galton, *Hypothyroidism: The Unsuspected Illness* (New York: Thomas Y. Crowell Company, 1976), 204, 205.

Chapter 18

1. B. O. Barnes, "Basal Temperature versus Basal Metabolism," *Journal of the American Medical Association* (August, 1942): 119:1072.

2. J. C. Scott, Jr., and Elizabeth Mussey, "Menstrual Patterns In Myxedema," *American Journal of Obstetrics and Gynecology* (1965): 90:161.

3. M. S. Gold, H. R. Pearsall and A. C. Pottash, "Hypothyroidism and Depression: The Causal Connection," *Diagnosis* (December, 1983): 77–80.

BIBLIOGRAPHY

Adams, Ruth. *The Complete Home Guide to All the Vitamins.* New York: Larchmont Books, 1976.

Barnes, Broda O. and Charlotte W. Barnes. *Heart Attack Rareness in Thyroid-Treated Patients.* Springfield, Illinois: Charles C. Thomas, 1972.

————. *Solved: The Riddle of Heart Attacks.* Fort Collins, Colo.: Robinson Press, Inc., 1978.

————. *Hope for Hypoglycemia.* Fort Collins, Colo.: Robinson Press, Inc., 1978.

Barnes, Broda O. and Lawrence Galton. *Hypothyroidism: The Unsuspected Illness.* New York: Thomas Y. Crowell Co., 1976.

Bodansky, Meyer and Oscar Bodansky. *Biochemistry of Disease.* New York: The Macmillan Company, 1940.

Bricklin, Mark. *The Practical Encyclopedia of Natural Healing.* Emmaus, Pa.: Rodale Press, Inc., 1976.

Davis, Adelle. *Let's Get Well.* New York: Harcourt Brace & World, Inc., 1965.

Elwood, Catharyn. *Feel Like a Million.* New York: The Devin-Adair Company, 1952.

Fredericks, Carlton. *Psycho-Nutrition.* New York: Grosset & Dunlap, 1976.

Fredericks, Carlton, and Herman Goodman, *Low Blood Sugar and You.* New York: Constellations International, 1969.

Mandell, Marshall, and Lynne Waller Scanlon. *Dr. Mandell's 5-Day Allergy Relief System.* New York: Pocket Books, 1980.

Masor, Nathan. *The New Psychiatry.* New York: Philosophical Library, 1959.

Newbold, H. L.. *Dr. Newbold's Revolutionary New Discoveries About Weight Loss.* New York: Rawson Associates Publishers, Inc., 1977.

Passwater, Richard. *Supernutrition for Healthy Hearts.* New York: The Dial Press, 1977.

Philpott, William H., and Dwight K. Kalita. *Victory Over Diabetes.* New Canaan, Connecticut: Keats Publishing, Inc., 1983.

Pinckney, Cathey, and Edward R. Pinckney. *Do-It-Yourself Medical Testing.* New York: Facts on File, 1983.

———. *The Fallacy of Freud and Psychoanalysis.* Englewood Cliffs, N.J.: Prentice-Hall, Inc., 1965.

Pinckney, Edward R., and Cathey Pinckney. *The Cholesterol Controversy.* Los Angeles: Sherbourne Press, 1973.

Staff of *Prevention. The Encyclopedia of Common Diseases.* Emmaus, Pa.: Rodale Press, Inc., 1976.

———. *The Complete Book of Vitamins.* Emmaus, Pa.: Rodale Press, Inc., 1977.

Randolph, Theron G., and Ralph W. Moss. *An Alternative Approach to Allergies.* Toronto, New York: Bantam Books. 1982.

Rubin, Herman H. *Glands, Sex, and Personality.* New York: Wilfred Funk, Inc., 1952.

Williams, Roger J., and Dwight K. Kalita. *A Physician's Handbook on Orthomolecular Medicine.* New York: Pergamon Press, 1977.

Williams, Roger J. *Free and Unequal.* Austin, Tex.: University of Texas Press, 1953.

———. *Biochemical Individuality.* New York: John Wiley & Sons, Inc., 1956.

INDEX